The Management of the Aging Process

By

Louis N. Chude

Disclaimer

Table of Contents

The Concept of Age

"Age is just a number." Isn't this one of the most famous sayings that we all hear time and again? As clichéd as it sounds, it is very true. We are only as old as we believe ourselves to be. Having said that, we can't ignore the fact that as we grow older, our health declines, making it essential to monitor our health and managing the aging process well is quite important for us. We get to live only once. So, it is on us to live a healthy and prosperous life.

The truth is that age doesn't spare anyone. We all have to go through different stages of life. It's a cycle that is the same for everyone. The only thing that differs is how we choose to grow older. To live a quality life, we need to focus on our health. Aging gracefully is important. There are so many older adults who just ignored their health, and today, they are living compromised lives. A little care and attention could have helped them avoid this.

While no single key explains the concept of aging, there are several studies that have been done that talk about slowing down the aging process. These studies show that to slow the aging process down, we need to focus on our physical and mental selves and become better versions of ourselves.

Most people around us fear aging. Why?

They fear nearing the end. They fear being dependent on others. They fear facing health problems. They fear being a burden on others. They fear not being able to support themselves financially. The truth is that we all have to grow old. There is no way we can escape this stage of life. So now that we have accepted it as a reality, the best way forward is to deal with the process to the best of our abilities and create a plan that allows us to live a healthy and prosperous life.

Ashton Applewhite talked about aging in her TedTalk. She said, "Aging is not a problem to be fixed or a disease to be cured. It is a natural, powerful, lifelong process that unites us all."

It's something so relatable, isn't it?

Aging is most definitely not a problem. It is us who make it a problem. It won't seem as hard if we just accept it and plan for it.

The biggest problem I see today is the idea of eternal youth. The media sells the idea of eternal youth to us on a daily basis. It is something that is helping so many industries thrive too. However, there is no such concept as eternal youth. We all have to age at some point in time. The sooner we accept it, the sooner we can start planning for it. We must reject the fear and celebrate evolution.

Through this book, I want to shed light on how we can all manage the aging process. All of us are getting older with each passing day. If we plan and start to manage the process, we will stop fearing the idea of growing old and will definitely embrace it.

Important Statistics

Globally, the number of people aged 65 years and above increased by 6 percent from the year 1990 to the year 2019. Projections show that this number will rise by 16 percent by 2050. With the number of older people increasing globally, it is more important than ever to learn how to manage the aging process.

Statistics also show that Japan has the highest number of old-aged people.[1] However, the healthcare facilities there are also up to par, which means that the country is fully well-equipped to deal with any health issues. But that is not true for most countries. Most countries do not have the kind of platforms available to deal with the burden of health crises, which implies that we must take care of our health and ensure that we age healthily.

Managing the aging process is not as hard as it seems. All that it requires is willpower and determination. What we need to realize is that our health comes first before anything else, and we need to make sure that we take care of it. We get to live only once, and it is on us to make the most of it as well.

---

1 PRB, 2022. *Countries With the Oldest Populations in the World.* [Online]. Available at: https://www.prb.org/resources/countries-with-the-oldest-populations-in-the-world/#:~:text=Asia%20and%20Europe%20are%20home,at%20just%20under%2022%20percent.

The Role of Nutrition

Healthy aging is a topic that is widely discussed in the modern age. One of the most crucial factors that affect healthy aging is nutrition. As the adage goes, *"You are what you eat."* Whatever you take inside of you is what gives you strength and energy, which is what eventually allows you to lead a healthy life as well.

As you grow older, your body changes, too, so you must alter your eating habits accordingly. As you grow older, your systems become slower, so you need to eat just right to give your body the energy it needs to sustain itself. This certainly doesn't mean that you eat in excess quantities. Doing so negatively impacts your health. Ensuring healthy aging also reduces financial and social burdens, enabling you to live a quality life.

When it comes to healthy eating, your preferences become secondary. However, it also doesn't mean you can't eat what you like. It just means that you must be more mindful of what you take in and how it affects your body.

Here are a few things you need to follow when it comes to nutrition.

- You need to eat foods that give you ample nutrients without taking in too many calories since extra calories will only lead to weight gain, which is the last thing you need in this process. This means that you can eat fruits and vegetables in abundant quantities. That will keep you healthy. Also, pick ones that are bright in color since those are the most packed with nutrients.

- Try to eat whole grains like oatmeal and brown rice. These can give you all the energy that you need.

- You also need to focus on making your bones stronger. Often, people tend to fall when they are older, which leads to their bones getting fractured. To avoid such unfortunate incidents, it is imperative that you focus on your calcium and vitamin D intake. You can always take supplements here. However, it is best to focus on consuming food rich in these nutrients. For example, you can take low-fat or soy milk to help your calcium intake.

- You must also eat seafood and lean meats to give you all the nutrients your body needs. Other foods include poultry, eggs, beans, nuts, and seeds.

- You must try to avoid foods with empty calories. These include chips, candies, sodas, and other baked goods. Such food items don't give you any nutrients. The only thing they do is give you extra calories and make you fatter.

- It is also wise that you pick foods that are low in cholesterol and fat. Fats from animals are usually saturated fats which aren't good for you. High cholesterol is bad for your heart and is what ultimately leads to heart attacks as well. Try to avoid processed fats as much as you can. Foods that are rich in processed fat include margarine, bakery foods, and fried foods. While it is acceptable to indulge in them once in a while, make sure that you are wise about the choices you make daily.

- Another very important thing you need to consider is an intake of enough liquids. They keep you from getting dehydrated. The best way to do that is to ensure that you keep track of the amount of water you have in a day.

Nutrients Your Body Needs

Here are a few nutrients your body needs the most as you age.

- *Calcium and Vitamin D*

  Adults over seventy years of age often face issues with their bones (News, 2016). This is why you need to focus on ensuring that you get enough Calcium and Vitamin D from a young age to develop healthier bones over time. Like I mentioned above, it is always smarter to pick natural foods that are filled with these nutrients. However, if you still lack these nutrients, you can also opt for other supplements to help fulfill your nutrition needs.

- *Vitamin B12*

  Adults over fifty usually aren't able to absorb as much vitamin B12 (Wong, 2015). Foods that are rich in vitamin B12 include cereal, lean meat, and seafood. However, it is best that you get yourself checked, and if you still feel that you don't have enough of this vitamin, you can get supplements that can help you.

- *Dietary Fiber*

  Eating fiber-rich foods helps lower the risk of heart disease and type 2 diabetes. It also allows for healthier bowel movements, a common problem in older adults. Foods rich in fiber include bread, cereals, beans, peas, and lentils. Vegetables are also a great source of fiber.

- *Potassium*

  A lot of older adults face issues with high blood pressure. For that, adequate potassium is imperative. Foods that are rich in potassium include fruits, vegetables, and beans. However, you also need to limit your salt intake to manage your blood pressure. If you want to add more flavor to what you are eating, try to do that with other herbs and spices, but limit your intake of salt.

- *Folic Acid*

You need some folic acid to help you stay healthy. Too little of this nutrient in your body is a leading cause of anemia and increases the risk of babies being born with a defect, making this nutrient much more important for women than men. Fruits and vegetables have very high quantities of folic acid in them.

- *Magnesium*

When you grow older, you are much more prone to catching viruses and falling sick easily. For that, you need to make sure to have a very strong immune system. To ensure this, you need magnesium in your body. It also helps you with around three hundred different physiological processes. Not only that, but it helps heart health and your immune system too. Whole foods are the best source of magnesium in your body.

- *Healthy Fats*

One of the most common misconceptions is that fat is bad for your body; this is a wrong perception. While you don't need extra fat in your body, you surely need some fat to help you get the energy you need. That said, you only need healthy fat in your body. Foods with healthy fat include nuts, seeds, avocados, and vegetable oils.

Foods to Avoid

Now that you know what foods you need, here is a comprehensive list of foods you need to avoid.

- *Alcohol*

  A lot of older adults have an alcohol addiction. This is one of the worst things you can do to your body. Try to avoid alcohol as much as you can. Too much alcohol can lead to different types of cancers and can also damage your liver to a great extent. Apart from that, it can also lead to further problems like diabetes, high blood pressure, stroke, and so on. So try to limit your alcohol intake as much as you can. If you are suffering from an addiction, then you take things one step at a time and try to overcome this problem.

- *Red Meat*

  You must try to avoid red meat as much as possible. It is one of the leading causes of high cholesterol. Not just that, but it also leads to an increased risk of different types of cancers. As an alternative to red meat, you can have other lean meats like poultry or fish. Those are good for you and aren't even heavy meats. Research suggests that red meat consumption is also related to Alzheimer's. Since forgetfulness is a common problem among adults, it is smart to avoid red meat as much as possible. If you like red meat, try limiting your consumption as much as possible.

- *Processed Foods*

  Natural food is always the best since it doesn't have any additives. Processed food, on the other hand, has a lot of sodium, which harms your body more than you can ever imagine. We need only a very small amount of sodium to function normally on a daily basis. Excess sodium means you are at a higher risk of developing heart disease and other cardiovascular complications.

- *Excess Sugar*

  Your body doesn't need all of that excess sugar. It only increases your chances of developing diabetes. So you must limit your sugar intake as much as you can. When preparing your food at home, the ideal way to reduce sugar is to reduce it by around 30% on average. That can make a significant difference and contribute greatly to your healthy lifestyle.

- *Deep-Fried Food*

  When you have deep-fried food, you only take in excess fat, which is not what you need. It only adds calories without giving you any energy.

Having said all of that, it is completely understandable that you feel like eating certain things at certain times, which aren't all healthy; this practice is completely normal. We all have cravings, and it is completely understandable if you sometimes feel like indulging in them. But what you need to be mindful of is that such indulgences need to be occasional. On an everyday basis, you must have an eating schedule. You must stick to it to increase your chances of leading a healthy lifestyle.

Now that you understand the role that nutrition plays, you must start your journey of healthy eating today. Remember to take it one step at a time. It isn't something that will happen overnight but is an ongoing process.

Melina Jampolis, a very famous nutritionist, talked about the important role of nutrition. She said, "The best piece of advice when it comes to New Year's resolutions, whether your goal is to eat healthier, lose weight, exercise more or stress less, is to lose the all-or-nothing mentality."

She also talked about the importance of setting more achievable goals. "Set smaller interim goals or milestones on the path to your larger goal (and write them down in a journal to look back on your successes for extra motivation), and don't let a few setbacks throw you completely off track. Small, practical changes over time add to big results." [2]

Ways to Start Your Health Journey

I have already mentioned why it is important to start small and take things one step at a time. But it can be quite hard for those who are foodies or those who haven't been watchful eaters their whole lives. Here are a few tips that can help.

- *Slow Down*

When you eat, slow down. Enjoy your food and count your blessings while at it. This will prevent you from overeating. Studies have shown that fast eaters are much more likely to eat more and gain weight as compared to slow eaters (Fegerberg, 2021). Slow eating can reduce the number of calories that you consume over time. Apart from that, it also allows you to chew your food properly, aiding the digestion process.

- *Always Carry a Water Bottle with You*

I have already stressed the importance of consuming water in sufficient amounts. But when you carry a water bottle with you, you don't just drink water when you're thirsty. The bottle in your hands acts as a reminder for you to stay hydrated constantly. Not just that, but drinking water often also helps you feel full, preventing you from eating more than you need to. So it is a win-win situation for you.

- *Shop With a List*

When you go grocery shopping, don't go without a list. Write down all you need, and then make sure you get only that. When you have healthy things in the house, you wouldn't want

---

2 Berger, S., 2021. *10 Pieces Of Expert Nutrition Advice For 2022.* [Online] Available at: https://www.forbes.com/health/body/expert-nutrition-advice/

to eat out more. It increases your chances of eating healthy and cooking homemade meals. Impulse buying is also a very common problem. You need to stay away from it to be able to stay healthy.

- *Bake Your Food*

It is always best that you bake your food. Grilling and frying mean you use oil, which isn't good for you. So the best option for you is to bake your food. This helps you stay healthier. Broiling and poaching are also good options. But try to stay away from frying as much as you can.

- *Replace Your Favorite Fast-Food Restaurant*

Who doesn't like fast food?

However, as you grow older, it is best that you replace that with some other healthier options.

Stress Mitigation

According to the American Medical Association, "It has been verified through scientific exploration that more than 80 percent of all diseases are due to stress and strain that originate in the mind and reflect on the body" (Judson, n.d.).

With the fast-paced lives that we all live today, stress is unavoidable. We all have a certain degree of stress, which is also the leading cause of most diseases. But what really is stress? Simply put, it is the body's reaction to anything that disrupts our physical and mental equilibrium. When the body goes into a fight or flight state, we undergo stress.

A research study on stress in older adults showed that life stress is inversely related to physical and mental health. A total of 134 people aged 50 to 85 were part of this study. The study showed that mindfulness helps manage stress well.[3]

The negative impacts of stress, especially for elderly people, are disastrous. They are the leading causes of many medical problems that later affect the quality of life.

Here are a few negative effects that stress can have on one's health:

- Increased heart rate

- Increased muscle tension

- Higher blood pressure

- Rapid breathing

- Slowed down the digestive system

3 de Frias, C. M., & Whyne, E. (2015). Stress on health-related quality of life in older adults: the protective nature of mindfulness. *Aging & mental health*, *19*(3), 201-206.

- Weaker immune system

- Lack of sleep

With that being said, it is evident that stress only leads to the quality of life going down majorly. When we age, our systems get much weaker, so the last thing that we need is stress. For healthy aging, one of the most important things is to reduce stress in our lives. We need to make a more conscious effort to do this to live a quality life.

But before that, it is important to understand the important symptoms that can tell you that you are undergoing stress.

Symptoms of Stress

Here are a few common symptoms of stress that can tell you that you need to do something about it immediately.

Physiological Symptoms

- Insomnia

- Waking up with nightmares every other night

- Loss of appetite

- Palpitations

- Frequent urination

- Muscle pain

- Tiredness

Emotional Symptoms

- Anxiety and fear

- Difficulty when trying to concentrate

- Frustration

- Restlessness

- Forgetfulness

If you feel like you have any of these symptoms, then you must take action immediately to mitigate this.

Stress Management

Before you start with stress management, you need to understand that it is almost impossible to eliminate stress from your life. What you can do is minimize it as much as possible.

Furthermore, it is also essential to understand that there is no one way to deal with stress. It affects everyone differently, and different stress management techniques work for different people. First, you need to understand yourself and your requirements. Then you need to tailor the methods according to what works for you.

Here are a few stress management techniques that can help.

- **Mindfulness**

Mindfulness is one of the best ways that you can deal with stress. It can help you reflect and focus on the good as much as possible. It allows you to enjoy the moment you are in without worrying about anything else.

To practice mindfulness, start small. Spare ten to fifteen minutes of your day for mindfulness. This can be any time that you like. Sit or lie down in a quiet place and practice deep breathing. Try to breathe away all the negative energy and inhale positivity from your surroundings. Make a conscious effort to let go of all that is bothering you. When practicing mindfulness, try to be grateful for everything you are blessed with.

YouTube also has a lot of videos on mindfulness and how you can practice it. Not just that, but there are also many apps for older adults which help with guided meditation. This way, try to make mindfulness a part of your daily routine. You will see how much it helps you calm down in no time.

- **Exercise**

Exercising has many benefits. Not only does it help you improve your physical health, but it also helps you with your mental health. You can engage in any type of exercise that you like. It can be walking, tai chi, water aerobics, yoga, or anything else that works for you. The most important thing is for you to enjoy your workout. It should help you feel healthy, both inside and outside.

As an older adult, you might not be able to exercise as rigorously as you once used to. Fret not. What matters is that you need to be doing something to keep your body moving. Not only does regular exercise help you with your health, but it also helps you sleep better, hence allowing you to be more productive throughout the day.

Research shows that exercising releases endorphins, which help you maintain a positive attitude. So make an exercise routine and stick to it to maintain your health.

- **Have a Sense of Community**

Old age is often accompanied by feelings of loneliness and glumness. To overcome that, you must have a social circle. This can be anyone whom you like to hang out with. Your significant others can help you calm yourself down. It is also known that when you speak to others about what is troubling you, you can naturally calm yourself down in a much better way.

Happiness is greatly dependent on warm relationships. A sense of community helps you build these warm relationships, thus increasing happiness and reducing stress.

- **Nutrition**

I have already stressed the importance of healthy eating in the chapter earlier. You must ensure that you eat well and that your body gets all the nutrients required to function effectively. When that happens, you tend to feel much more energized.

When you eat well, you get all the nutrients your body needs for optimal functioning. This also, in turn, affects your mental health and your stress levels.

- **Avoid Tobacco and Nicotine Products**

Many people tend to use tobacco for stress management. The effect that it has on the body is quite the opposite. It makes you more stressed and also reduces blood flow and breathing. Try to avoid these products as much as possible.

For some people, it is an addiction, which means they cannot let go of it altogether. If you are addicted to tobacco products like cigarettes, try to quit this habit. Take it one step at a time, and you will surely be able to make some progress. It will take time and seem hard, but with ample effort, you will surely get what you want.

- **Reduce Triggers of Stress**

Many things trigger stress, and they vary from person to person; find out what triggers you and work on it. Sometimes, our lives are filled with too many to-do lists in too little time. This means that this excess demand can place too much pressure on us. You need to find out what triggers you and then reduce that. Manage your time well, and set priorities to achieve the most in the least amount of time.

- **Set Realistic Goals**

Often, we tend to set far-fetched goals for ourselves, which are too hard to achieve. This puts more pressure on us, which means that we can't get things done in the right way. Failure to accomplish what we want can make us feel insufficient, affecting our minds negatively.

To avoid this, we must set goals we know we can achieve. Remember not to be too hard on yourself. It is alright to falter once in a while and not be able to give your best to something. You don't need to push yourself to a point where it becomes stressful. This is where realistic goal setting takes precedence. When you have realistic expectations, you can naturally be at more ease.

- **Do The Things You Like**

Apart from your routine chores, you must set aside time to do things you like. Again, there is no formula for this. It can be anything that you enjoy. If you like sewing, knitting, or even painting, take time out for that. It can help you calm down and enjoy the little things in life. It also makes you feel much happier. Even if you have a very busy schedule, take some time out to do these things. Nothing helps you unwind better than that.

- **Solve Cognitive Puzzles**

Solving different cognitive puzzles can help provide mental stimulation, which serves as brain exercise, helping you calm down and increase your focus levels. You can get these puzzles from the local store and spend some time doing these brain exercises daily. It is, in fact, a very helpful distraction that can help you remain calm.

- **Prioritize Yourself**

Sometimes, being too giving can also be a problem. You need to learn how to say no. If something is bothering you, making you feel overburdened, or not allowing you to focus, then you need to learn to say no to all these things. Prioritize yourself and make yourself your number one. Whenever you feel overwhelmed with all that is happening around you, remind yourself of your worth and tell yourself that you are strong enough to get over anything you want. This way, you can have healthy self-esteem as well.

When you start doing these things, you learn a lot about yourself. You probably will find out what works for you and what doesn't. Not just that, but you will also understand how to start small and build yourself up. Remember that it is one step at a time. Slowly but surely, you will get there.

Not all of these stress management techniques might work for you. You need to find out what helps you and how it allows you to live a better life. That way, you can start your journey, and slowly you will be able to get there.

Routine Medical Checkup

Old age brings with it greater chances of health problems. You are much more likely to get diabetes and heart disease as you age. Some of these conditions don't show symptoms unless the disease progresses greatly. For this reason, it is important to get routine medical checkups done at your ease.

Unfortunately, older people don't want to get these checkups done. They're very reluctant and tend to take it very lightly, without really understanding what it can lead to.

When you go for your routine checkups, the doctor will ask you many questions to help him determine your health condition and advice you based on that.

Here are a few reasons why it is important to get routine medical checkups done.

- **Reduced Chances of Getting Sick**

When you get older, recovering from a mild fever also seems to take forever. When you get routine checkups, you can take preventive measures beforehand, which means you can greatly reduce your chances of falling sick. The doctor can tell you what you need to avoid and how that can help. Doing so will allow your health to improve over time.

- **Get Up to Date on Screenings**

Your doctor will also recommend checkups that will help you stay on track with the type of treatments you need. So, for example, the doctor will tell you all the vaccines you need to get to avoid flu, pneumonia, and so on. It is always better to be safe than sorry here. As the adage goes, prevention is better than cure. You should also remember that medical treatments are expensive, so being proactive can help you save money later.

- **Gain Control Over Chronic Conditions**

If you have a chronic disease like diabetes or any heart-related problem, it only worsens with time unless you're extra careful. Regular doctor visits can easily find the day-to-day care you need to help you deal with your condition. The doctor can also check the medicines you are taking and whether or not any changes are needed to help you later. This way, you can have greater control over any type of chronic condition and can slowly but surely recover from it.

- **Makes You More Educated**

Every time you visit the doctor, you learn more about the disease you suffer from. Not just that, but you also learn so much more about yourself. This helps you stay informed and also helps you understand your health conditions, which is imperative as you grow older.

- **Saves Money**

On the face of it, it might seem like you're spending more money on routine visits to the doctor. But in actuality, you are saving up more. How is that?

By taking preventive measures, you are saving yourself from any other diseases you might get later in life. In the case that you get certain diseases, you will have to end up spending much more on the treatment. So, in the long run, you end up saving money.

- **Build A Relationship with Your Doctor**

At this stage in your life, you need to have a good relationship with your doctor so that they can help you and make you a priority whenever needed. With regular visits to the doctor, you can surely build a very long-term relationship with him, which is exactly what you need. If you build that level of trust with your doctor, it will be much easier for you to go to them whenever you need to. Not just that, but you can speak to them about anything that you might need help with- for example, alcohol addiction. It can help you better understand yourself, and you will know what to do in case further health-related problems arise.

- **Increases Your Chances of Living Longer**

When you get regular checkups done, it becomes possible for you to detect any issues that have arisen with your body. The earlier the issues are detected, the sooner they can be cured, which means you live healthier lives. This increases your chances of living longer, allowing you to live a more fulfilled life.

If you have crossed the age of fifty, then it is of utmost importance that you get yourself checked regularly. This isn't an extra burden on your pocket but is more of a necessity that helps you live longer, allowing you to detect any issues early. This means that the chances of getting cured are also much higher.

You need to understand that your health is your biggest blessing. The sooner you understand this, the better it is for you. Therefore, taking care of your health should be your priority.

This brings us to the next question: What is all included in your routine checkup?

What Should Be Included in a Routine Checkup?

During your regular checkup, the doctor first looks at your history and then evaluates your current health based on how you feel. Here is what the doctor will look at:

- Your medical history

- Your family history of diseases

- Things you are allergic to

- Your list of regular medication

- Your vaccination

- Your history of screening for various diseases

Preparing for Routine Checkup

To ensure that your routine checkup works out as planned, you must be prepared for it. You need to be able to answer the doctors' questions well to ensure that there are no errors.

Here are a few things you should do before your routine checkup.

- Make sure you have all your medical information with you- any reports you need to show the doctor, your insurance, old health records, or anything you think the doctor needs to see.

- If anything has changed since the last time you visited the doctor, you need to remember that and let your doctor know about it.

- Make sure you are fully updated with all the medicines you are taking. You need to have a list of those so you can also tell your doctor about them.

- If you have special needs, you also need to tell your doctor about those.

Talking To Your Doctor

You must keep a few things in mind when speaking to your doctor. This is important to ensure that your visit is successful.

- Make sure that there is open communication between you and your doctor. You should be able to speak to your doctor about anything without shying away from it. This person is responsible for ensuring you are healthy and well, so you must build that rapport with him.

- Have a list of questions that you want to ask him. This can be anything that you are unclear about or anything that is bothering you. Remember that no question is a stupid one. You should be able to ask your doctor anything without worrying that he won't answer you or will judge you.

- If you are unclear about anything, your doctor says, be sure to ask him again, so you don't remain confused. This is imperative to ensure that your treatment is up to the mark.

- While your doctor is talking, take notes. It always helps to remember important things in case you forget something later.

- Ask your doctor what their preferred mode of communication is for a follow-up. This is important to ensure that you can contact them in case of an emergency and also so that you can schedule a follow-up appointment accordingly.

- If you don't agree with something, your doctor says, tell him that so that he can tell you alternate ways of doing it. Remember that it is all about you being comfortable with your doctor.

- Many people avoid topics like sex and drug abuse when talking to their doctor. You don't need to worry about that. Remember that the doctor is there to help you. However, he can only help you when you are open about everything and choose to talk about it.

Ideally, you should try sticking with one doctor for a long time because they know your entire history. You can also build a relationship with the doctor, which is important to ensure all issues are cleared out there and then.

Screening of Age-Related Diseases

When you grow older, your immune system naturally becomes weaker. This means you are more likely to be affected by any type of disease. For this purpose, it is important to screen for age-related diseases. Regular screening ensures that you detect any abnormalities early on and that you get them treated at the soonest. It is a part of preventive healthcare, a field that is being explored continuously. The main idea is to ensure that any diseases are detected well before time so that the chances of curing completely are much higher.

So what is a screening test?

A screening test is done to detect any potential health disorders in people with no symptoms of the disease. The main idea is to reduce the risk of the disease by taking all the necessary preventive measures. Not just that, but the focus is on ensuring that if there are any lifestyle changes needed, then the patient should be made very well aware of those as well.

Common Age-Related Diseases

Here are a few age-related diseases. As you age, you have a greater chance of developing these diseases.

- **Cardiovascular Disease**

This disease is one of the most common causes of death in older adults. This includes the risk of congestive heart failure, artery diseases, hypertension, and atrial fibrillation. It becomes much easier to tackle if diagnosed at an earlier stage. The most common form of coronary artery disease is when the arteries get blocked, and blood cannot flow to the heart easily. This can even lead to heart attacks happening.

Here's a breakdown of the symptoms, causes, interventions, preventive measures, and types of tests for early detection of cardiovascular diseases:

Symptoms	Causes	Emergency Intervention	Preventive Measures	Medical Checkup for Early Detection
• Chest pain • Breathlessness • Fatigue • Dizziness • Swollen limbs • Faster palpitations	• Family history of the disease • High use of tobacco • High use of alcohol • Greater consumption of sugar and fat • High cholesterol • High blood pressure • Diabetes	If the patient cannot manage their pain or gets unresponsive, family members urgently need to take the patient to an emergency.	• Have a healthy diet • Focus on exercising • Stop smoking • Take medicines for diabetes regularly • Try to remain in a healthy weight range based on your body mass index • Don't leave out any medicines	• Blood tests • Stress tests • Ultrasounds • Coronary angiogram

- **Cerebrovascular Disease**

This is more commonly known as a stroke, which happens when blood doesn't reach the brain due to disruption in the blood vessels. Brain cells that don't get ample oxygen tend to die very quickly. There are mainly two types of strokes. These are ischemic strokes and hemorrhagic strokes. These two are the leading causes of death in older adults. In some cases, these strokes can even cause severe blockage or rupture.

Let's take a look at the symptoms, causes, interventions, preventive measures, and types of tests for early detection of cerebrovascular disease:

Symptoms	Causes	Emergency Intervention	Preventive Measures	Medical Checkup for Early Detection
•Excessive headache •Inability to speak well •Extreme confusion •Dizziness •Nausea •Vomiting •Misinterpretation of information	•Stress •High use of tobacco •High use of alcohol •Poor diet •High cholesterol •High blood pressure •Diabetes	If the patient starts shivering excessively and this gets worse at a very fast pace, then emergency intervention is needed	•Have a healthy diet •Focus on exercising •Stop smoking •Lose excessive weight •Control high blood pressure	•Blood tests •Physical checkup for the whole body •Echocardiogram •Cerebral angiogram •MRI •CT scan

• High Blood Pressure

High Blood pressure is when the blood in your body puts great pressure on your arteries. This leads to an increase in blood pressure. On the other hand, when you are at rest, your blood pressure may become too low. Neither is good for you and can cause serious issues like heart problems and kidney problems.

The symptoms, causes, interventions, preventive measures, and types of tests for early detection of high blood pressure are given below:

Symptoms	Causes	Emergency Intervention	Preventive Measures	Medical Checkup for Early Detection
• Excessive headache • Chest pain • Difficulty breathing • Urine in the blood • Fatigue • Vision issues	• Stress • High use of tobacco • High use of alcohol • Genetics • Extra salt in food • Lack of physical activity	There is no emergency situation in blood pressure. It is a silent killer, which is why it needs to be managed over time slowly	• Have a healthy diet • Focus on exercising • Stop smoking • Sleep well	• Echocardiogram • Blood tests • Ambulatory monitoring

- **Cancer**

Cancer is a disease that kills thousands of people every year. Age is one of the biggest risk factors for cancer. It develops when abnormal cells begin to grow in the body. According to research by the American Cancer Society, 77% of cancers develop in people over the age of 55. When screened earlier, the chances of getting cured are naturally much higher.

*There are several types of cancers, each with its own symptoms, causes, and preventive measures. Each needs to be looked into separately.

That said, here's a summary of the symptoms, causes, emergency interventions, preventive measures, and medical checkups for early detection of three of the most common types of cancers.

- ## **Prostate Cancer**

Symptoms	Causes	Emergency Intervention	Preventive Measures	Medical Checkup for Early Detection
• Problems when urinating • Blood in urine • Erectile dysfunction • Bone pain	The causes aren't specific. However, it is related to the mechanism of your DNA	If a person stops responding, then there is a dire need to see a doctor	• Eat healthy food • Regularly exercise • Increase vitamin D intake • Remain active sexually	• Prostate-specific antigen test

- ## **Breast Cancer**

Symptoms	Causes	Emergency Intervention	Preventive Measures	Medical Checkup for Early Detection
• Breast lumps • Breast thickening • Irritation of breast skin • Redness of nipples	• Age • Family history • Exposure to radiation • Genetics	If a person has immense pain in the breasts, then they need emergency care	• Eat healthy • Remain physically active • Breastfeed children as much as possible • Reduce smoking	• Mammogram • MRI

- ## **Cervical Cancer**

Symptoms	Causes	Emergency Intervention	Preventive Measures	Medical Checkup for Early Detection
<ul><li>Irregular vaginal bleeding</li><li>Pain during intercourse</li><li>Pelvic pain</li><li>Extreme pain when on period</li></ul>	<ul><li>Long-lasting infections</li></ul>	If a person stops responding, then they need immediate care	Regular screenings and tests	<ul><li>Pap test</li><li>HPV test</li><li>Biopsy</li><li>X-ray</li><li>CT scan</li></ul>

Type 2 Diabetes

Diabetes is a chronic problem that is related to the way that your body makes use of glucose in the body. Type 2 Diabetes is also one of the health problems that are more common in older adults and is also the leading cause of heart problems and kidney failure.

Here's a summary of its symptoms, causes, emergency interventions, preventive measures, and tests for early detection:

Symptoms	Causes	Emergency Intervention	Preventive Measures	Medical Checkup for Early Detection
<ul><li>Greater urge to urinate</li><li>Excessive fatigue</li><li>Numbness in different body parts</li><li>Extra weight loss</li><li>Increased hunger</li></ul>	<ul><li>Extra weight</li><li>Lack of exercise</li><li>High blood pressure</li><li>Family history of diabetes</li><li>Polycystic ovaries syndrome</li></ul>	If a patient feels drowsy and faints, then family members need to take them to the emergency	<ul><li>Reducing intake of carbohydrates</li><li>Eating a diet high in fiber</li><li>Limiting intake of alcohol and tobacco</li><li>Losing extra weight</li></ul>	<ul><li>Glucose screening tests</li><li>Glucose tolerance test</li><li>Random blood sugar test</li><li>Fasting blood sugar test</li><li>HBA1c test</li></ul>

- **Parkinson's Disease**

This is a neurological disorder that causes tremors in the body. Around 75% of Parkinson's cases begin after age 60 (Philippe Rizek & Jog, 2016). Researchers believe that there are a lot of genetic factors that also affect the chances of getting this disease.

Here's a breakdown of the symptoms, causes, interventions, preventive measures, and types of tests for early detection of the disease:

Symptoms	Causes	Emergency Intervention	Preventive Measures	Medical Checkup for Early Detection
• Intense mood changes • Depression • Urinary infections • Skin problems • Constipation • Difficulty speaking	• Genetic factors • Environmental factors like exposure to toxins	Sleep attacks and aggravation of motor symptoms can happen	• Eat fresh food • Ensure that there is ample Vitamin D3 in your food • Exercise regularly	• The doctor checks for different nervous system changes • There are no specific tests for this

- **Dementia**

This is a disease in which ideal brain functioning stops. It can result in memory loss, drastic mood changes, confusion, and also difficulty when communicating. Alzheimer's disease also counts as part of dementia. Most health experts believe that the incidence of dementia is a natural part of the aging process.

Its symptoms, causes, emergency interventions, preventive measures, and tests for early detection include:

Symptoms	Causes	Emergency Intervention	Preventive Measures	Medical Checkup for Early Detection
• Confusion • Memory loss • Unable to speak fully • Feeling lost • Repeating things over and over	• Poor diet • Excessive alcohol usage • Smoking • Depression • Genetics • Cardiovascular issues	If a patient is unable to breathe well, then they need to be taken to the emergency room	• Eat a balanced diet • Exercise regularly • Limit alcohol intake • Keep blood pressure under control	• Cognitive tests • Brain scans • Genetic tests • Psychiatrist evaluation

- **Chronic Obstructive Pulmonary Disease**

This disease leads to reduced airflow into and out of the lungs, which leads to the thickening of the lungs on the inside and extra mucus being produced. This is more common in adults over the age of 65. While this condition cannot be cured, it can be prevented greatly if detected in time. Constant exposure to tobacco smoke is one of the leading causes of this disease.

Here are the symptoms, causes, emergency interventions, preventive measures, and tests for early detection of this disease:

Symptoms	Causes	Emergency Intervention	Preventive Measures	Medical Checkup for Early Detection
• Difficulty breathing • Cough • Excessive passing of gas • Mucus development	Smoking	If a patient is unable to breathe well, then they need to be taken to the hospital emergency at the soonest	Stop smoking	Spirometry

- **Osteoarthritis**

This is one of the most common forms of arthritis. As people age, their chances of getting this degenerative disease become higher. In this disease, the joints tend to swell up and, thus, cause pain. While this disease cannot be fully cured, it can be managed well if the right medication is taken. Changes in our lifestyles, like exercising and eating healthy over time, might also be needed.

The symptoms, causes, emergency interventions, preventive measures, and tests for early detection of osteoarthritis include:

Symptoms	Causes	Emergency Intervention	Preventive Measures	Medical Checkup for Early Detection
• Increased pain in the joints • Extra stiffness in joints	• Genetics • Injuries • Extra pressure on joints	If a patient is unable to breathe well, then they need to be taken to the hospital emergency at the soonest	• Keeping the right posture • Losing eight • Exercising regularly	• Joint fluid analysis

- **Osteoporosis**

This is a disease in which bone mass lessens, which causes the bones to become much weaker. As you age, you have a greater chance of getting this disease. Vitamin D deficiency is also one of the leading causes of this disease. When your bones become weaker, you tend to have greater chances of hip fractures, which can be quite problematic for older adults, restricting their movement. This is also one of the leading causes of death in older adults, typically after a year of injury.

The symptoms, causes, emergency interventions, preventive measures, and tests for early detection of osteoporosis are as follows:

Symptoms	Causes	Emergency Intervention	Preventive Measures	Medical Checkup for Early Detection
• Weak nails • Height loss • Frequent bone fractures	• Lack of calcium • Having an unhealthy diet	If a person has compression fractures, then they need to see a doctor as soon as possible	Eat foods rich in calcium and vitamin D	• Bone density test

- **Cataracts**

This is a disease in which cloudiness appears in front of the lens of the eye, disrupting vision. While there are other causes of the disease, too, like smoking and diabetes, age remains the top cause. Many people need to have cataract surgeries when older so that they can get them removed.

If left untreated, it tends to make the vision blurred. Doctors usually recommend surgery to most patients for this disease.

The symptoms, causes, emergency interventions, preventive measures, and tests for early detection of cataracts include:

Symptoms	Causes	Emergency Intervention	Preventive Measures	Medical Checkup for Early Detection

				Retinal exam
• Double vision • Blur vision • Halo around lights	• Injury • Aging	• If a patient is unable to see well over time, then they need to get checked for it immediately	• Manage other chronic health issues • Have a healthy diet • Reduce alcohol intake • Quit smoking	

• Hearing Loss

Hearing loss is also one of the most common age-related diseases. There is tiny hair in the ear that processes sound.

With age, these tend to deteriorate, which is what causes issues when processing sound. This means that it can lead to simple changes in hearing and problems with distinguishing certain consonants.

The following are the symptoms, causes, emergency interventions, preventive measures, and tests for early detection of hearing loss:

Symptoms	Causes	Emergency Intervention	Preventive Measures	Medical Checkup for Early Detection
• Needing to hear in loud volumes • Difficulty understanding certain words	• Exposure to loud noise • Ototoxic medications • Head injuries	If a patient is unable to hear at all, they need to be taken for medical examination	Don't expose yourself to extra noisy activities	Audiometer tests

While aging is not a problem, the diseases that come with it can cause many issues. This means you are more likely to get these diseases as you grow older. For this reason, you need to ensure that you get regular screening done to detect any illnesses much earlier on. Screening helps you identify any diseases at an early stage, which means that the chances of you being able to get rid of these are also much higher.

Financial Aspects of Maintaining Health

There is no denying the fact that healthcare has become very expensive in the current day and age that we live in. That said, it is not an expense we can cut down on. Come to think of it; our health is the biggest blessing we have been bestowed with. To age peacefully, we must look after our health.

Healthcare costs differ greatly based on where you live. Countries with the most affordable healthcare in the world include Brazil, Costa Rica, Cuba, Japan, and Malaysia (Tips, 2020). In comparison, the country with the most expensive healthcare is the United States of America. To maintain your health, you must surely consider the financial aspect of the same and take action accordingly.

Here are a few things that you should consider when it comes to the financial aspects of maintaining health. These can help you look at things in more detail and plan accordingly.

- **Plan Ahead**

One of the most important things you need to consider is planning ahead of time. You must understand the importance of planning ahead. When you retire, that is the time when you count on your savings the most.

Understand that the chances of you needing medical care later in your life can be much higher, so you should have a saving plan in mind, specifically for healthcare. Put aside a certain amount every month, specifically for healthcare later on. It will help you later in life if you have a medical emergency to attend to.

- **Routine Screenings**

The importance of routine screenings and checkups has already been stressed earlier. You must get routine screenings and checkups to detect any health issues early on. Doing that can save a lot of money since you are aiming for preventive care instead of treatment, which can be quite expensive.

- **Take Care of Yourself**

Always remember that your health comes first. You can't afford to be careless about it. So always prioritize yourself. Have a healthy meal plan and always exercise to keep yourself as fit as possible. The fitter you are, the lesser the chances of you getting sick. We all have to age someday, so we might as well plan that things unfold for us in the best possible way.

- **Health Insurance**

Healthcare insurance is one of the most important things you need to consider when it comes to managing the financial aspects of healthcare. This is covered in great detail ahead.

Health Insurance

Health insurance is a contract in which the insurer pays for a person's healthcare costs. For this, you have to pay a certain monthly premium based on your selected package. Nowadays, it is highly important to get health insurance for own self. Medical emergencies can cost quite a lot. They can punch a massive hole in your pocket if you aren't insured. At this moment, health insurance comes into action and plays its role.

Types of Health Insurance

There are two broad categories of health insurance. These are individual cover and family cover. The type you get depends entirely on what you are looking for, whether or not a family member has a chronic illness and the number of family members you have.

⇒ Individual cover- this is when the insured sum is for one particular person. This type of insurance is most suited if a person needs constant medical treatment.

⇒ Family cover- this plan covers the whole family. The sum insured can be used regardless of who needs medical treatment.

Why Do You Need Health Insurance?

Health insurance is one of the most critical aspects of financial planning. Unfortunately, many people don't feel a dire need to get health insurance. We don't realize that with general healthcare costs skyrocketing, it is essential that we get coverage. Here are a few reasons why health insurance is vital.

1. **Rising Medical Costs**

Medical inflation is now becoming a huge issue with new technologies emerging. This implies that we must get coverage if we wish to protect ourselves. Most people end up spending most of their savings on medical emergencies. This is the last thing that you want, right?

2. **Rising Lifestyle Diseases**

Chronic diseases like diabetes and respiratory issues require regular medical treatment. However, with these diseases now becoming more common in older adults, getting treatment for them can be quite expensive. For this reason, getting health insurance is imperative. It allows you to manage these diseases well by getting the right medication without spending a fortune.

3. **Family Protection**

Medical emergencies can occur at any time. With health insurance, you can protect your family. This is especially true for the older adults in the family, who have greater chances of falling sick since they have a weaker immune system. You will always be stressed about medical treatment and its costs without appropriate health coverage.

4. Preventive Care

You might overlook minor health issues without insurance coverage, which quickly escalate into bigger issues. Preventive care is always the best option, allowing you to detect the problem as it arises. The chances of curing the disease are also much higher when that happens. If you have health insurance, regular screening and tests aren't an issue.

Factors to Consider When Finding an Insurance Company

With so many different insurance companies, picking one can seem quite daunting. Here are a few tips to help you find a good insurance company.

1. Reputation

The most important part is to find out about the insurance company. You can do a background check to see how long the company has been in business. You can also check all the services they provide and the reviews people have given. This can clarify the position of the company and can help you understand how good the company is. With several companies, it is important to run a background check and compare them. This helps you make a very well-informed choice.

2. Type of Policy

Everyone has different requirements. Before selecting an insurance company, you first need to check the type of policies they have. Remember that it is essential for you to get adequate health coverage. Based on their offerings, you can check their policies and see which one matches your needs.

1. Affordability

The monthly insurance you have to pay is a fixed expense each month. Based on the type of policy you want, you can compare the monthly premiums you must pay. You must keep your budget in mind here. After all, managing expenses is becoming more challenging, given the rising inflation rates. You should pick the policy that seems the most reasonable and gives the highest coverage.

2. Hospitals Covered

Most insurance companies have a specific list of hospitals on their list. You need to make sure that you check that list first. If you are a frequent traveler, it is even more important for you to thoroughly go through this list to find out about their list of global hospitals.

3. Renewal Policy

Some insurance policies need to be renewed after every few years. So you need to check the renewal age based on whom you want insurance for. Purchasing a life insurance policy is ideal if you are an older adult. It helps you save yourself from hassle later on.

4. Claim Process

It is extremely important for you to go through the claim process. Unfortunately, some companies have a very complex claim process, making it very tedious. Look for a company with simplified procedures, allowing you to get the best customer service.

5. Pre/Post Hospitalization

There are a lot of tests that need to be done before you get hospitalized. After the procedure, there might be a lot of medications that you may need too. So you must also check the insurance plan to see if it covers all aspects. The more coverage it provides, the better it is for you.

6. Waiting Time

Many insurance providers have high waiting times before you can make a claim. This only makes it more inconvenient for you to make a claim. Before selecting a company, find out about their waiting times - the shorter the waiting time, the more appealing the insurance provider.

Make sure you consider all of these factors before making the right choice.

When Should You Purchase Health Insurance?

A common misconception that people have is that you only need to buy health insurance later on in life. This is not the right approach. The ideal time to buy health insurance is in your twenties. This is because you should begin planning for your old age when you are young. That said, medical emergencies can occur at anytime, so if you are covered, it will help you avoid the stress of such incidents.

If you are older and haven't yet purchased health insurance, you should do it soon. It is never too late to invest in your health! Remember that your health is your biggest blessing.

Social and Family Interactions

For older adults, mental health is as important as physical health. However, we don't see much attention being given to mental health in people as they grow older. It is very common to see older adults in social isolation. Either it is because of their lack of willingness to socialize with others or because they don't have the means to stay connected at all times.

When older adults socialize, it makes them healthier and happier, giving them a sense of purpose in their life. It is important that they remain busy doing something productive to ensure that there are no feelings of loneliness. Many older adults fall prey to depression because they spend too much time alone. This is the root cause of all evil. Socializing ensures brain activity, allowing them to live happier and healthier life.

Benefits of Social and Family Interactions for Older Adults

Here are a few benefits of social and family interactions for older adults.

- **Sense of Belonging**

The biggest advantage is that it gives them a sense of belonging. It makes them feel like they have a purpose they want to fulfill. When they listen to others and share their opinions, they feel like others value them, and that is when they get the motivation to continue investing in those relationships. This enriches their lives and makes them feel much more productive as well.

- **Keeps them From Getting Bored**

At an older age, there isn't much to do in life. Most elder people spend their time alone and tend to get bored. However, with interactions with their family and other members of their social circle, they keep themselves busy and enjoy their time. This is very important to ensure they remain happy and fulfilled.

- **Improves Health**

The health benefits of social and family interactions for older adults are many. It helps them battle feelings of loneliness. Research has also shown that it reduces the risk of Alzheimer's disease and lowers blood pressure (Zhaoyang et al., 2021). It keeps their brain functioning well too. All of this only adds to the quality and their lives. Not just that, but it also increases the chances of longevity.

- **Reduces Stress Levels**

Who doesn't have stress in their lives?

Especially for older adults, stress has become much more common. With so much spare time on hand, they tend to worry about things a lot, even if they aren't remotely related to them. High-stress levels lead to poor health conditions, causing depression and anxiety. Continuous interaction with others distracts them, which eventually helps reduce stress levels.

- **Keeps them happy**

More than anything else, it is vital that older adults are happy and content in their lives. For this, they mustn't have feelings of loneliness. Social interactions allow them to feel more valuable, reducing levels of anxiety and stress, in turn keeping them happy and improving the quality of their life.

Overall, it can be seen that all of these benefits allow older adults to remain happy and content with their lives. It allows them to understand things better and focus on living a positive life.

Tips to Form Social Connections

For older adults, forming social connections can seem like a task. Some even think it takes too much effort from their end. Here are a few useful tips that can help with that.

- **Join an Exercise Group**

There are many exercise groups that older adults can join. These groups can help them work out alongside other people of their age, which gives them motivation. Not just that, but they can also socialize with the other people in that group, allowing them to expand their social circle.

- **Speak About Your Discomfort**

A lot of older adults aren't comfortable meeting many people daily. If that is the case with you, you should be open about it and speak to someone who can guide you. They will help you figure out what to do to form social connections.

- **Connect via Technology**

Technology has enabled us to become more connected with the world around us. While there is no substitute for face-to-face connection, it just isn't possible for some people, especially those who are immobile. In this case, you can remain connected to others through social media platforms like Facebook or Instagram. That is better than completely isolating yourself from others. When older adults isolate themselves, their minds wander to places they shouldn't. They keep thinking about things they shouldn't think of, which tends to depress them.

- **Make Neighborhood Friends**

Connecting with neighborhood friends is a great idea. When you live close to someone, you can easily meet each other and make convenient plans. This can help you remain connected to others around you, allowing you to build lasting bonds with others.

- **Make Phone Calls**

If you have friends who live far from you, call them once in a while to check on them and see what they are up to. It can help you remain connected with them. It will also make them happy to know that you still think about them and want to maintain that bond with them. This helps them stay by your side long-term and eventually makes your social circle larger.

- **Volunteer**

Older people often have a lot of spare time on hand. So they can make the most of their time by volunteering. There are many available options. For example, they can volunteer at other old age homes and speak to others of their age. They can also volunteer at orphanages and help young children in need. Not only does this help them stay connected with society, but it also gives them a feeling of being useful. This is, in fact, extremely important to make older people feel productive. Giving back to society is a great idea since it gives this feeling of self-satisfaction, which is great!

These useful tips can benefit older adults in forming social connections. When older adults remain connected with others, it helps them understand things much better. It can also help them feel good about themselves and their lives.

Forming stronger connections with family is as important as forming social connections. Most older people tend to cut themselves off from their family members and usually like to stay in their zones. This practice often makes them feel lonely.

Family members should make sure that they keep asking older adults if they need anything. They should spend ample time with them and talk about different things. Even if they seem hesitant to speak, the family members should make an effort from their end. This can help them feel much more at ease.

Tips to Form Stronger Family Bonds

Here are a few ways that stronger family bonds can be developed.

- **Understand Each Other's Issues**

The key to forming a stronger bond is understanding that each of us goes through different things in life. Family is one's backbone to lean on. So, the first thing you need to do is understand each other. If you have older adults living in your house, understand them and their needs. If they have health issues, be supportive and show that you care. We all have to age someday, so we should treat our older family members the way we want to be treated when we grow older.

- **Nip the Evil in the Bud**

Whenever an issue arises between family members, try to address it right at the moment. If you prolong it for some other time problem only worsens. Communicate with each other and understand where the other person is coming from. Understand what the issue is and try to solve it instantly. When you do that, the chances of a healthy relationship becoming even stronger are much higher.

- **Set Realistic Expectations**

Most people tend to have very high expectations from family members. And when they can't fulfill them, it only disappoints and thus weakens the relationships. Don't let that be a hindrance in your relationship. Understand that everyone has different responsibilities, and they might not always be able to provide you with their best. When you set realistic expectations, the chances of disappointment become minimal, allowing you to build stronger connections.

- **Respect Each Other**

The foundation of all relationships is respect. You can only form stronger and healthier bonds if you respect each other and understand that boundaries exist. If someone does something wrong, tell them so in a respectful manner. Understand that everyone has free will, and you can only exercise your will on yourself. Most problems arise because family members start dictating to each other. When you try to control someone else's actions, it will only make them feel uncomfortable and caged to a great extent, compromising your relationship. Don't let that happen at any cost!

- **Be Honest**

It is also essential to be open and honest with each other. If there is something that you feel a family member has done that they shouldn't have, speak to them about it and tell them how it made you feel.

- **Spend Time With Each Other**

You must spend time with each other. This means that you must explore common interests and spend time with each other doing things you love. This will only allow you to make the most of your time together and have a good laugh while at it too. This allows family bonds to grow stronger.

- **Make Meal Time Together a Priority**

Set a certain time when you can have meals together. This is extremely important to build that connection with your family. No matter how busy you are, take some time to have at least a single meal with your whole family. This promotes healthy discussion and allows family members to sit together and catch up, speaking about their respective days. These wholesome conversations allow everyone to understand each other and connect deeper. It also helps you get to know your family members much better.

- **Do Daily Tasks Together**

As a family, there is a lot that you can do together. This includes things like cooking and cleaning. This way, you can get to spend so much quality time together. It also promotes that connection between family members.

- **Support Each Other's Interests**

Know what your family members like to do, and then support them in getting a step closer to their dreams. You will see how much that impacts their life. When your family knows that you have their back no matter what, they will hold you closer and make sure they are there for you when you need them.

These tips can allow you to form stronger family bonds. For older adults, these family bonds are extremely precious as these tips can improve the quality of their lives.

Long-Term Factors Affecting Health

Your health is something you need to invest in and hence is based on multiple factors. We see many older adults above the age of seventy doing many things that even fifty-year-olds can't do. Why is that so?

It is because they have invested in their health and are much fitter. This happens because they take care of themselves since the beginning and thus reap the benefit later in life.

Excess fatigue, sleeplessness, and drowsiness generally accompany old age, drastically reducing the quality of life. So, when you are young, you need to be extra careful about your mental and physical health. When you do that, you will see how much better off you are as compared to the rest of the people your age.

Here are a few long-term factors affecting health. If you start focusing on them early, it can help you improve the quality of your life. There are some you can have full control of, while there are others you cannot do anything about. Either way, you must make as much effort as possible to exercise discipline from an early age.

The Social and Economic Environment

This is something that you do not have complete control over. Of course, social mobility is possible, but even that is hard.

- **Income**

The amount of money you earn significantly affects how you can take care of yourself. You can surely spend much more on yourself if you earn a decent income. You can invest in quality healthcare and focus on eating more whole foods, which is eventually great for you.

- **Education**

If you are highly educated, you are naturally much more well-informed about things. This means that you can make much more planned and thought-out decisions for your life, which allows you to be healthier. For example, you can make smarter food choices based on your caloric needs. Not just that, but you can also focus on consulting the right people when needed. You also understand the importance of exercising when you are educated. When given two options, you can surely choose the one that seems best after weighing out the pros and cons of each.

- **Social Support**

You can understand yourself much better based on the society you live in. Social support can help you become much healthier mentally too. Factors like stress and anxiety can be dealt with more easily when you have support from those living with you. It can help you make wise decisions based on what the other people around you think. It also gives you something to lean on in times of need.

- **Employment/ Working Conditions**

You spend a significant percentage of your day at work. This tends to affect the way you live your life significantly. It holds true for your physical health as well as your mental health. For example, those who work in mines have a significant risk of developing different diseases because of the harmful substances they are exposed to. Not just that, but their life is in danger too.

Hence, the quality of their life is much poorer. Similarly, suppose you have a toxic working environment where people are backbiting about each other, and there is very little constructive activity happening. In that case, it can affect how you think and process things, eventually leading to stress. I have already touched upon the effect of stress in life and how it can be more detrimental than we think.

So if you think your workplace has a toxic culture, understand why there is a dire need to make that shift. Understand why that switch is imperative for your wellbeing. People often stick to toxic workplaces for several reasons, like money, social status, etc. While these are important factors to consider, make the smarter choice, bearing in mind what is more important to you.

To understand this better, let's consider what a toxic workplace culture entails. It includes failure to include people at work equally, disrespect, unethical behavior, unneeded politics, and so on. All of this can lead to anxiety, panic attacks, and depression.

Research has shown that a toxic workplace is ten times more likely to drive workers away (Robinson, 2022). When employees don't feel valued, they don't like to stay and look for better opportunities.

Healthy Behaviors

This includes your nutrition and level of activity every day. I have already focused on how important it is to have a balanced diet. When you have a habit of eating healthy, you give your body all that it needs to function well. Your diet needs to include all food groups so that there is nothing you miss out on. Try to take as much natural food as you can. While packaged ready-to-make meals can seem like a very convenient option today, they can deprive you of the required nutrients to live a more fulfilled life.

For those looking to eat healthily and remain fit, a meal plan is a great idea. It can help you stick to a routine, allowing you to eat from all food groups. You can even get in touch with a nutritionist who can assess your health and check your goals. Based on that, they can guide you about the food you should eat. This can surely help you remain much healthier.

Apart from that, it also includes your activity level. Time and again, health experts have stressed the importance of remaining active. Many older adults complain of aching joints. Why is that so?

Apart from other underlying health conditions, it is also a result of low activity levels. When you sit idle, doing nothing, it affects your body in unimaginable ways. Try to remain as active as possible. This doesn't mean you need to go to the gym every day, even if you don't like to. Try to indulge in any physical activity you can from a very young age. This can be anything at all that you like to do. For example, if you like cycling, walking, or swimming, just do that. Anything that helps you keep active should suffice.

Here are a few other tips that can help:

- Do all your daily chores yourself, like cooking and cleaning. This is something that also helps you remain extremely active at home.

- Take breaks from long hours of sitting at one go. Maybe you could go for a round after every hour at work. Not only will that help you stay active, but it will also help you refresh your mind.

- Try to get all of your groceries yourself too. Walk to and from the grocery store near your house, and you will see how that helps you stay active.

Healthcare

Based on where you live, quality healthcare is a significant factor that affects your overall wellbeing. This includes regular doctor's visits, screenings for diseases, and so on.

In countries with high-quality healthcare, there are regular doctor visits and appropriate screening. This practice increases the chances of any issues being detected early on. The right type of care depends on the quality of the outpatient clinics, hospitals, and public health departments. In countries where healthcare is a priority, doctors tend to call patients for routine visits. If you live in a part of the world where healthcare isn't considered very important, then this is something you need to take care of on your own so that you can get the care that you require.

If you want to take care of your health and see continuous improvement, then you need a lifestyle change. Unfortunately, many people switch back and forth between different periods of drastic changes, which does nothing but harm the body more than you think. For example, many people struggling with weight issues tend to try fad diets for a short time and then fall back into their cycle of unhealthy eating. This periodic cycling only tarnishes their system more, making them more prone to these unhealthy habits. This is one of the worst things you can do to your body.

If you genuinely want to care for your health, you must focus on a lifestyle change. Focus on changing yourself for the better. If you are a foodie, then make a routine for yourself. Maybe you could eat your greens on the weekdays and then indulge on the weekends. It will help if you change the entire way you live and work on yourself so that being healthy becomes a natural part of your lifestyle.

For example, that one hour of daily activity should not seem like a chore. It should not seem like you are doing something out of compulsion. Instead, start enjoying that one hour. Breathe out all the negative energies and focus on how much this is helping you improve your lifestyle. You will see how much you look forward to that one hour of your life when you only focus on your health. This physical activity session can be anything that you like to do. Just do it with all your heart and see how much you love it then.

Remember, the key to improving your health this way is through self-love. You need to love yourself enough to make those changes that seamlessly blend into your life and don't seem like extra chores for which you must make an effort. When you do that, you will see yourself slowly transforming into the healthiest version of yourself, which is eventually what you want for yourself, ultimately.

Self-Love

Self-love is all about making yourself the center of your world. You must focus on yourself and love yourself more than anyone else. This surely doesn't mean that you become selfish. It only means that you understand yourself and your body and then work towards improving.

Here are a few tips that can help you love yourself more. When you love yourself, anything you do for your health doesn't seem like extra effort. It only seems necessary.

- **Listen to Your Body**

If your body is telling you something, listen to it. If you feel tired and think you are sleep deprived, get in those extra hours of rest. You need it!

If you think you can walk that extra mile, do it. Listen to your body, and you will see how you will be able to do wonders in life.

- **Take the Idea of 'Perfect' Out of Your Mind**

There is no such thing as perfect. We are all humans, and we all make mistakes. The sooner we understand that, the better. Understand that there is no way you can be 'perfect' because that state is not achievable and does not exist. Do what your body allows you to do. If you think you need to see a doctor because of something that is bothering you, do it.

- **Don't Take Unsolicited Advice**

In today's times, many people tend to give advice even though you didn't ask for it. They don't even know anything about you but consider themselves more knowledgeable than anyone else.

When anyone gives you unsolicited advice, just listen to what they have to say, but don't take it seriously.

No one knows your body and mind better than you do. So either listen to yourself or your doctor, who knows your medical condition better. Remember that your health comes first, so you don't have to please others but have to take care of yourself first. Make yourself a priority!

- **Set Realistic Expectations**

Understand that you are human. You need to set realistic expectations. When you expect more than you can achieve, it only leads to setbacks and disappointment when you cannot get there. So you must set achievable standards from day one so there is no disappointment later on. You are your own hero. Understand that and accept that. You will see how your life will become so much better once you do this.

- **Stop Comparing Yourself to Others**

We live in a very competitive world, meaning cutthroat competition exists. So naturally, we tend to compare ourselves to others. We need to understand this- *We all are different.*

Our bodies are different, our goals are different, and our health conditions are very different too. So stop comparing yourself to others around you. It will only bog you down, making you feel like you aren't good enough. So that is the last thing you should be doing. It is detrimental to your mental health too. The only healthy comparison you should be making is between you yesterday and you today. That will help you focus on self-improvement, which is exactly what you need to do.

Your journey is yours alone. Comparing yourself to others can be counterproductive and can lead to ill feelings like jealousy. So make sure you never do that.

- **Allow Yourself to Make Mistakes**

More often than not, we tend to be too hard on ourselves. We don't allow ourselves to make mistakes, which is why we sometimes tend to be unforgiving. So learn that making mistakes is alright.

We all make mistakes, and that is how we learn. These mistakes help us grow into better versions of ourselves. Of course, the pressure to not fail is unavoidable. But try to make a conscious effort to remember that making mistakes is normal. It is what eventually helps you learn and grow. Your life is a journey where learning takes place at every step. So understand that, and embrace it.

No one is perfect, so stop trying to set unreal benchmarks. When you falter, get back up and learn from that. Try to grow as much as you can. Your mistakes aren't failures but opportunities that help you grow and make solid progress each day.

- **Remember to Have Fun**

With our packed schedules, we fail to have fun. We don't understand what it means to make time for the things we like to do. Understand how important that is for growth, wellness, and mental health.

Having fun doesn't necessarily mean going out of your way daily to make elaborate plans. It means enjoying the little moments and making them count the most. For example, if you look forward to that one cup of coffee in the evening after your walk, make sure never to skip it. If it adds that fun element to your life, do it. Never miss out on it because you need fun to add that feel-good factor to your life.

- **Practice Gratitude**

One form of self-love is to practice gratitude. When you do that, you see the things you should be thankful for. It helps you see all that God has given you without even asking for it.

Gratitude enables you to focus on the good in life, which is ultimately very important since it helps you understand things and gives you more clarity. Set aside five minutes of your day to count your blessings. It enables you to see how you're better off than so many people, making you feel good about your life.

Having a gratitude journal also helps since it allows you to jot down all that you have in life to be thankful for. Try to write down at least one thing you are genuinely thankful for every day. You will see how much that helps you down the road. The best time to do this is in the mornings, as it allows you to start your day with gratitude. This practice increases your chances of having a good day ahead too.

- **Acknowledge Oppression and Trauma**

If you have gone through anything negative in life, try acknowledging it and coming to terms with it. When you do that, you learn to deal with it in a much better way too. Blocking out your thoughts can make you feel caged. You also end up internalizing everything, which is far from good for your mental health.

Instead, acknowledge the bad, accept how you feel, and understand that it was a thing from your past. Remember that you now have to focus on the times that are yet to come. You will see how much that helps you. Dr. Gooden, a mental health counselor, spoke about acknowledging ill feelings.

According to him, most people tend to neglect their physical, mental, and emotional needs in an attempt to prove that they are worthy and deserve respect. Trauma survivors often internalize and blame themselves for what they experienced. They believe something is wrong with them, which is why someone chose to hurt them.

You need to understand that you don't have to be a victim of circumstance. Your life is a gift, and you are the one who has the power to make it work in your favor. So focus on improving your life as much as you can. You can even get help if needed.

- **Learn to Say 'No'**

Most of us can be too giving, which tends to drain us emotionally. Helping others is great, but so is setting boundaries. You need to learn to say no when there is already too much on your plate. Remember, you are important, too, so you need to make sure that you learn how to say no when needed. Only take up as much work as you can handle. When you take on more than that, it can be extremely challenging and can also induce great anxiety. When you know your boundaries, you will understand yourself better and be able to focus more on yourself than the people around you, which is ultimately very important.

When you are extraordinarily kind and selfless, saying no can be challenging. But try to inculcate this habit, and understand that you are doing this for yourself because you matter, and nothing matters more than your mental health and how you feel.

- **Know Your Strengths**

There are always some traits we have that help us outshine others. Know your strengths and put them to use so you can achieve your goals. When we achieve things in life, it can make us feel good about ourselves. So make sure to put your strengths to use in the right way. This helps inculcate positive feelings and helps you work on your goals. It is especially true if you're achievement-oriented, as you can use your strengths to build the life you want for yourself.

- **Let Go of Toxic People**

Your social circle plays a great role in the way you see things. When you surround yourself with toxic people, you also tend to have negative thoughts in your mind, which can transform you into a negative person too.

So, focus on the positives in life and let go of all of the people who are filling your life with negativity. Don't let them affect your life. How you process information depends greatly on the people you surround yourself with.

So, make sure you don't think twice before letting go of such people. Some people stick to the wrong people due to their fear of being alone. Remember that being alone is much better than being around the wrong people who drain you of all the energy you have.

So the sooner you let go of such people, the better it is for your mental health. When you let go of them, you will notice positive changes around yourself, which is what you need. Letting go of such people can be very liberating because they bring out the worst in you.

- **Take the Opportunities that Come Your Way**

Whenever you see a certain opportunity coming your way, grab onto it. You will see how much it helps you grow and move on to bigger things in life. To reach your goals, you need to focus on taking things one step at a time and make the most of any opportunity that comes your way.

Don't be frightened. Instead, take it on as something you need to do to build the life you want.

- **Look Past Your Physical Self**

In the age of social media, we are defined by our appearance. Filters on social media make everyone look flawless, which gives us a sense of indirect pressure to look our best. While there is nothing wrong with improving your appearance, it gets unhealthy when we have such far-fetched ideas of beauty.

Remember that no one is as pretty as these filters make them look. Also, no one shares the weak moments of their life on social media. So while you try to improve your physical self, also focus on your mental health and how you process information because that eventually affects how you feel things.

You will only be able to feel good and love yourself when you accept yourself the way you are and embrace every inch of your body. You are unique and beautiful just the way God has made you. So, focus on that. Let go of any thoughts of inadequacy and try to focus on who you are from within. Be comfortable in your own skin because that's when you'll shine brighter.

- **Stand Up for Yourself**

There's a fine line between being bold and being disrespectful. You must understand the difference and stand up for yourself when needed.

Understand that you need to be assertive when someone attacks you or blames you for something you haven't done. When you make yourself a priority, other people will automatically respect you too.

Remember that you're the only person who can stand up for yourself; no one will do it for you. You are your own hero, and the sooner you understand that, the better it is for you.

- **Understand That Not Everyone Will Like You**

Many of us try to seek validation from those around us. We try to get validation from those who barely know us. Understand that you are a person with numerous strengths and weaknesses. Not everyone will like you. There will be some who won't agree with most of the things you believe in. So don't let that affect you. Just as you don't like everyone around you, some won't like you either. So don't worry, and don't let that affect your feelings. You are different. You are unique. You are trying to be the best version of yourself. So focus on that, and don't let others bother you too much.

- **Ask For Help If Needed**

In trying to be self-sufficient, we sometimes don't understand how our bodies and minds are affected. If you feel like you need help, get help. We are human, and sometimes we struggle to get done with everything we have to do. This is especially true for those with multiple things to do in a day. Never shy away from asking for help. If you think you have too much on your plate, hire someone to help you with your chores. Remember that you need to make yourself a priority and focus on yourself more than anyone else to live a comfortable and fulfilled life.

Importance of Exercising

Most of us have repeatedly heard how exercising is good for us and that we should make time for it. Yet, we get lazy and try to avoid it. It is imperative to understand that exercising has countless benefits for healthy aging. Exercise is mistaken for holding heavy equipment or spending significant time at the gym. While in reality, it means any form of physical activity which allows you to stay as active as possible. It helps you maintain independence as you age.

Benefits of Exercising

Here are a few benefits of exercising that enable healthy aging.

- **Helps Prevent Disease**

When you remain physically active, you can reduce your chances of getting heart disease and diabetes. It is also great for your immune system since it allows you to fight off diseases much better. For people with disrupted sleep patterns, exercise is quite helpful. Since it tires you out during the day and allows for proper blood flow to reach your brain, you sleep well too. Exercising also helps fight off other diseases like hypertension and cholesterol.

- **Boosts Energy**

When you're younger, you feel healthy and active at most times. But when you age, you tend to feel more tired than usual. To fight this off, you can start exercising at an early age. This will help you stay active at all times. Not just that, but when exercising becomes a habit, it won't seem like something you must put a lot of extra effort into it.

- **Helps Improve Mental Health**

When you grow older, you generally don't have much to do. This can lead to loneliness and make you feel like you don't have much to look forward to. In this case, Exercising will be of best help. When you work out, your body releases chemicals that allow you to improve your mood and feel relaxed.

- **Strengthens Your Body**

Exercising helps you become stronger. We often see older adults tend to have frail bones and weaker muscles. When you exercise, you become stronger, allowing you to build your strength. It also allows you to slow down the loss of bone density that usually comes with age while helping you increase your muscle mass.

- **Reduces Risk of Falls**

Older adults tend to hurt themselves when they fall. Research has shown that working out helps you reduce your risk of falling since you become stronger. Falling is one of the worst things that can happen to older adults. It can even break bones, hampering physical movement later on, and exercising can help with that.

- **Helps Control Weight**

Obesity is the mother of all evil. It leads to numerous other diseases as well. When you control your weight, you are able to deal with all other problems well. Depending on your goal, you should try to burn as many calories as possible when exercising.

- **Keeps Your Skin Glowing**

Many people tend to have saggy skin as they grow older. Exercise helps you keep your skin looking fresh too. When you exercise regularly, your body produces natural antioxidants, which help you protect your cells. It also stimulates blood flow, allowing your skin to remain as fresh as ever.

- **Helps with Memory Function**

Many people feel like they cannot remember many things as they grow older. This is because their brain functions much more slowly. Exercising allows enough blood flow to the brain, which also helps improve memory. It enhances the brain's ability to process information. As a result, the hippocampus grows, allowing for better learning.

- **Reduces Pain**

Pain in different parts of the body usually comes with age. When left unchecked, it hampers functionality too. But when you make a habit of exercising regularly, this practice reduces pain significantly. As a result, your body becomes much better equipped to deal with pain too.

- **Increases Chances of Living Longer**

Exercising also increases your chances of living longer. This is because it promotes better health, which means that you do not have to struggle with different diseases. This not only increases your chances of living longer but also improves the quality of your life.

Most people struggle with exercise. They consider it too much effort to set some time aside during the day and engage in some form of physical activity. That said, you must remember that it is only as hard as you make it seem. You can start slow and become increasingly active over time.

For example, try to take the stairs instead of the elevator when going somewhere. This can allow you to stay active generally. Apart from that, try to spare an hour in the whole day to engage in some form of physical activity you like. This could include running, jogging, swimming, aerobic exercise, tennis, etc.

The catch is to make sure that you enjoy what you are doing. When that happens, you will automatically see how things become easier. You won't feel like it is an extra effort to spare that one hour of your day because you will enjoy every bit of your work.

If you are new to exercising and struggle to make it a regular part of your routine, then you can do a few things that can help.

Tips to Make Exercise a Regular Part of Your Routine

Here are a few tips that can help you take the first step. Once you take the first step, it will all seem much simpler.

- **Take Baby Steps**

Don't start with a heavy routine right at the beginning. Maybe you could start with something that initially won't seem too hard. For example, you could start with a thirty-minute walk in the neighborhood or cycle for a short while at your favorite time of the day. This will help you get your body in rhythm, which is exactly what you need. Once your body gets used to it, you can pick the pace and move on to something physically intensive.

- **Set Goals**

Goals give you something to look forward to. When you set goals, you can build your exercise plan according to them. For example, your goal could be to complete a five-mile run in a specific timeframe. This way, you can see how soon you get there and work towards increasing your pace. You can start with small achievable goals and work your way up.

- **Keep Track of Your Progress**

You get motivated when you see yourself making progress. This doesn't mean that you need to become a slave to the weighing scale. It only means that you track your progress in terms of how you feel as you get closer to your goals with each passing day. When you notice how exercising improves your life, you will surely want to keep going—set goals and a timeline to help you see how and when you can get there.

- **Make It Fun**

When you make your workouts fun, you will notice how it doesn't seem like extra effort. You can listen to your favorite music when working out or have a friend keep you company. This way, you will look forward to that one hour in the day when you work out.

- **Learn More About Fitness**

The world of exercise and nutrition is very vast and all the more interesting too. So, if you learn more about it and what it offers, you will surely see how your interest increases. You might even start trying out different routines.

- **Listen to Your Body**

Sometimes, we tend to ignore cues from our bodies, which makes the entire process much harder. So you need to listen to your body as much as you can. For example, if you feel like you get too tired when you swim, your body isn't liking it. The idea is to make your body more active instead of making you feel lethargic. So maybe you could then try other forms of workout. Listen to your body and see how it transforms slowly and gradually.

- **Seek Help from a Fitness Coach**

A specialist can help you chalk out a plan, making it much easier for you. You can get in touch with someone in the field. This can help you establish an exercise plan, making things easier for yourself. You will see how much it helps. You can even register for group classes. Then, when you work out with other people, you can motivate each other too.

- **Explore Your Options**

Exercising might initially seem very hard to you if you are a beginner and haven't worked out much. So you can explore all the different options you have. There are several forms of workout; make sure to check what works for you by exploring all of these options. This will help you understand yourself and your preferences much better.

Make sure you choose something you like so it doesn't feel like an extra effort. That said, you also need to be mindful of not getting lazy in this aspect because this can hamper graceful aging.

Types of Physical Exercise

There are several types of exercises that you can do, depending on what you like. You can even stick to three to four of these to make sure you get your body moving. Here are a few types of popular exercises for healthy aging.

Walking

Walking is one of the best forms of workout that helps you get those extra steps in. It is often recommended for older adults as it allows them to remain fit and only requires mild exertion. It is one of the most underrated forms of workout.

Dr. Matt Taneberg talks about walking as a form of exercise with great hemp benefits. He says, "Walking can be as good as a workout, if not better, than running. You hear of people 'plateauing' when they continue to do the same workout routine and stop seeing results. I see patients all the time that plateau from running; they will run the same distance, speed, and time, day in and day out. You need to constantly be switching up your exercise routine in order to get the maximum benefit for your health."

If you aren't one to invest a lot of energy into working out and want something with which you can remain consistent, too, then walking is one of the best forms of exercise for you. You can take some time out of your busy schedule and walk anywhere. You can go to the park if you wish, or you can even go to the nearest neighborhood. Walking can help you burn a lot of calories, depending on your goal. Having said that, it is not easy to start walking at a very fast pace initially.

Here are a few tips to help you get a head start when walking.

- Start slow. Walking for maybe fifteen minutes a day, whenever you find time, should work. This can help you get a headstart.
- Next, you can start off with brisk walking when you don't tire off that easily. Then, start picking up the pace once you get used to it. It shouldn't be too hard once you feel you have the energy you need.
- Maybe you could even find a partner who can make the process much more entertaining for you. You can just have a nice chat while you walk.
- Wherever you go, try to take the stairs instead of the elevator. You will see how much that will help you.
- If you get tired between walking sessions, it is always advisable that you take breaks. It will help you catch your breath, and you won't even find yourself too tired to function.

- Walking on the treadmill is also a good option for those who dislike walking outdoors.
- When you walk, make sure that you are wearing comfortable footwear. That will surely allow you to be comfortable when walking, which means that you can also walk long distances if needed.
- Whenever you walk, make sure to warm up and cool down before and after. This is one of the most important aspects since it helps set the tone too.

Yoga

Yoga is also one of the most popular forms of exercise. It focuses on strengthening your abdominal muscles and also allows you to focus on improving your core strength. This form of workout is highly recommended for seniors since it is a low-intensity workout, focusing more on body strength and stability.

Not only does it help with better balancing, but it also helps you calm down by focusing on slow breathing movements. You can even make your bones much stronger with yoga. It helps with mental relaxation too.

There are several yoga types that you can do, based on what suits you best. However, it all boils down to the poses that you can do. It needs to be tailored to your bodily needs. Here are a few things you can do when starting out.

- Find a yoga teacher. Someone who is experienced can teach you in a much better way. They can understand your body type first and then guide you accordingly. There are so many different classes that offer discounts, especially for seniors.
- You can even follow along on YouTube. There are so many channels that have comprehensive guidelines for

those who want to do yoga. Most of them have detailed step-wise instructions that can help.

- You need to find out which type of yoga works for you. That way, you will be able to understand your body better and will be able to do what is best for you.
- You can also start off with breathing exercises. Not only do these go well with yoga, but they also have a lot of other meditative benefits that can help.
- It is also extremely crucial for you to wear comfortable clothing. When you do that, you can do the exercises in a much better way. Make sure that the clothes are as breathable as possible.
- Also, get a yoga mat. This will help you start doing yoga at home.

Before you start, there are specific yoga poses you should have ample knowledge about. These include:

- Child's pose (Balasana) - This is a resting pose where you kneel on your shin bones and have your butt resting on your knees. You stretch out and have your forehead resting on the mat.

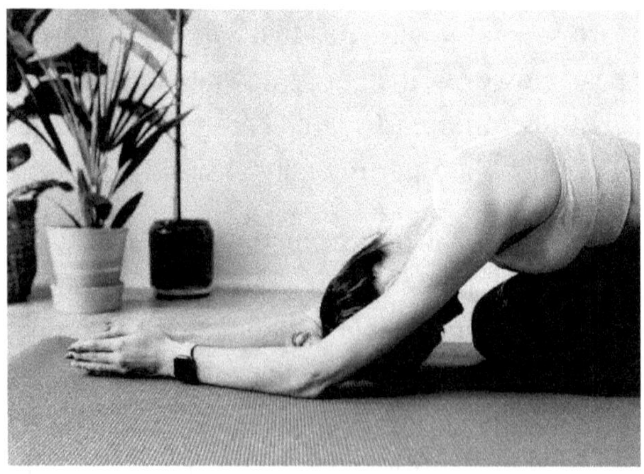

- Mountain's pose (Tadasana) - This is a standing pose in which you tighten your abdominal muscles.
- Standing forward pose - This is the pose in which you stand with your feet together on the yoga mat and bend forward to touch your knees.

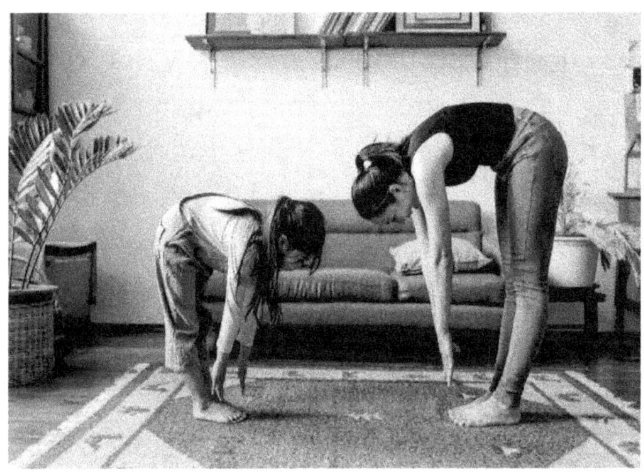

- Downward facing dog pose - In this pose, you stand with your toes on the ground and have your hips bent forward with your arms stretched out further—your chest points towards the ground.

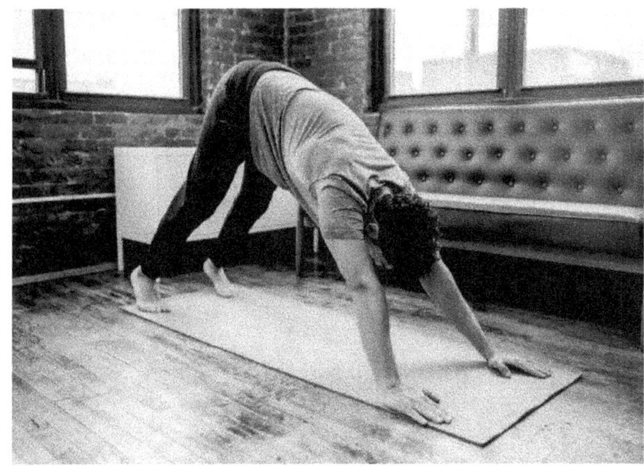

- Locust pose - In this pose, you lie on the yoga mat, belly down. You straighten your legs, placing your arms on the sides.

Swimming

Swimming is also one of the best forms of workout for older adults. Given that it has a comparatively low risk of injury and is also low impact, it is great for older adults. Swimming does wonders for heart health and also makes your muscles stronger. It also improves blood circulation, helping you calm down. It is very gentle on the joints, which means that it is a great form of workout that can help you remain active, allowing you to relax while at it. Swimming is one of the most recommended forms of workout that can help people remain active while adding to their flexibility.

More often than not, older adults usually refrain from working out because they are scared of injury. Not just that, but they are also scared of the fear of falling. Swimming can help deal with these concerns in the best way. Let's take a look at how:

- Water helps take the weight off the joints, so you won't feel too much pressure when working out.
- It helps your heart pump blood more efficiently. Improved circulation of blood leads to better health too.
- Swimming is also very healthy for the brain. It improves memory, concentration, and focus. Swimmers usually have better mental speed than others.
- Moving your body parts in water also means using greater force, which further adds strength and improves muscle strength.
- More than anything else, it helps improve your mental health since it allows you to focus on yourself and your well-being.

Water aerobics is also one of the best forms of workout that you can do in the water. It helps with building strength, alongside catering to other issues like those of arthritis and joint pain. Water brings natural resistance, which means that you will be able to work on building strength. Exercises that you can do underwater include aqua jogging, flutter kicking, leg lift, and arm curls.

Pilates

Pilates is one of the most popular forms of workout for older adults since it is low impact. It focuses on slow breathing, alignment, and posture. With moves solely based on your body weight, you can focus on developing core strength and improving flexibility. This is one form of workout specifically designed to help you build strength and improve your flexibility.

There are several benefits of Pilates for older adults.

- It helps build a stronger core. The idea is to help build strength and allow for greater control.
- It also helps focus on breathing movement, creating a calming effect.
- It helps correct muscle imbalances.
- There are several age-related problems like arthritis that it helps deal with too.

Here are a few Pilates exercises that are good for seniors.

Forearm planks- These are great for building core strength. Based solely on your core strength, planks help focus on your abs, helping build up your strength. You need to lie down on your stomach and position your elbows and feet straight on the ground. Then you need to lift your hips and hold the position for around thirty minutes before returning to the floor.

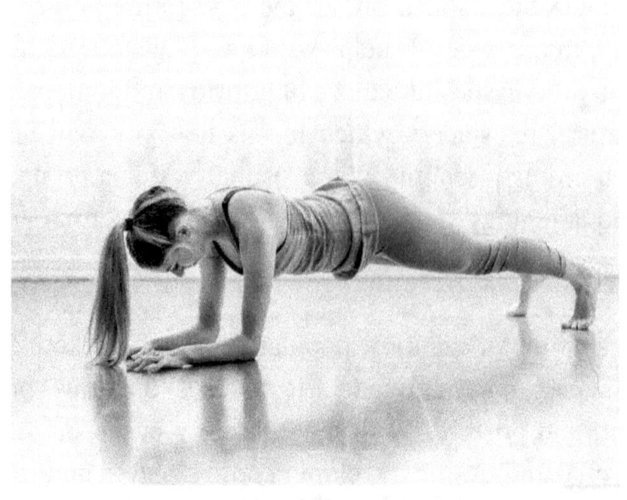

Bird dog- This pose is similar to the one above. The only difference is that one arm and one leg is lifted. This again engages your core fully and allows you to build your strength up. Then the same has to be repeated on the other side as well.

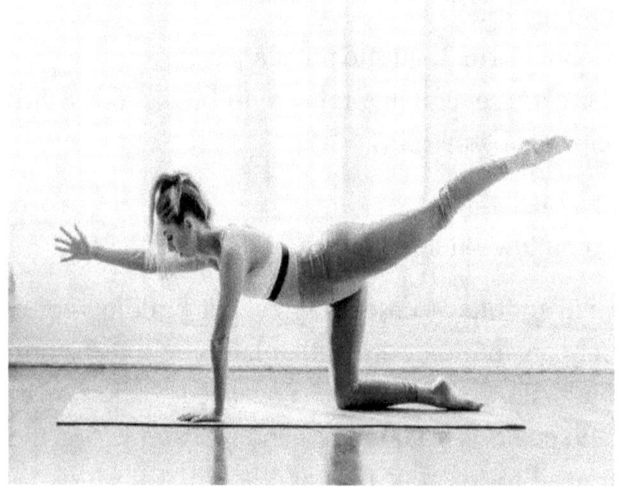

Mountain climbers- This is when you start off with a high plank and bring your knees towards your chest one by one. Then you keep switching. If you want your pulse to be higher, you must continuously keep doing this at a much faster pace. This engages your core and glutes fully, allowing you to build up your strength as much as possible.

Pelvic curl- This involves lying on your back with your knees bent, with your feet apart. Then you have to keep lifting your butt and holding for at least thirty seconds.

These are basic Pilates moves that help you build core strength.

Cycling

Many older people don't like the idea of sparing extra time and putting it into something like exercising. The idea seems pretty tedious to them, which is why they usually like to do something that is more exciting. Cycling is one such form of workout which can be quite entertaining. You can find people in your neighborhood and can go cycling with them. Not only does it help you remain healthy and fit, but it also allows you to have fun while at it.

Cycling helps you remain active and makes your immune system much stronger. All you need is a high-quality cycle, and you're good to go. An even better idea is to cycle to places where you need to go. For example, you can go to buy groceries as you cycle. That can help you save up on fuel expenses too. So if you're looking for a physical activity that also delivers other benefits, then cycling is your best option.

Strength Training

Strength training is a great idea for those looking to build greater strength and look fitter. Most older people don't opt for strength training because it seems too strenuous. However, it doesn't have to be. Strength training programs for older adults are designed in such a way that they target a few muscle groups. They also don't put any extra strain on lifting heavy weights.

If you opt for strength training, you must get in touch with someone who is an expert. A coach can help you design a plan more suited to your needs. They can help you identify what workouts are good for you and how much weight you need to lift, depending on your body weight and strength.

Now that you know all about the different types of physical activity that you can do, you must choose one that you think works best for you. The idea is to understand your body and your needs first before you pick something for yourself.

How Much Exercise Do Older Adults Need?

This is a question that many have. While there isn't one straight answer to this, the idea is to make sure that you keep as active as possible. If you can focus on working out every day of the week, then this would deliver the best results. But more often than not, that isn't really possible for older adults, who are often relatively low on energy. So, ideally, the target should be at least two to three days a week of working out. This can again be any form of workout that helps you remain active and allows you to improve your balance.

For beginners, it is always better to start slow and then build your way up. You can increase the intensity of your workout accordingly. You will slowly notice an increase in your stamina. What might seem very hard initially will slowly start to seem easier as you make some progress. Understand that this is a process that will take some time to develop. It would help if you worked hard and will see how much that helps you build your way up. You will slowly be able to build your stamina as well.

Safety Tips to Keep in Mind

While the benefits of working out are many, you also need to understand that there are several safety tips you need to bear in mind while at it. Remember that your health is most important, and if anything doesn't seem right at any point in time, you should know that it isn't working out for you. There is a specific time to test a particular exercise for your body; if the practice is not helping you, you must move on to the next.

- **Stop When You're Uncomfortable**

For example, if you start feeling dizzy or short of breath, you need to stop instantly and take a break. If you feel like your joints are swelling up, you need to consult a medical health practitioner as soon as possible, who can better guide you. You need to remember that you aren't suited for everything. Some things might suit you, while others might not. So if any workout makes you feel even the slightest bit uncomfortable, you need to stop.

- **Have Water**

When exercising, you need to make sure that you carry a water bottle with you at all times. It would help if you were extra careful about this during summers when the chances of getting dehydrated are much higher. You should sip water throughout your workout session.

This certainly doesn't mean that you gulp down an entire bottle of water before you begin working out. It just means that you keep a bottle with you and keep sipping some throughout the session. This will help you remain hydrated and full of energy throughout. However, you need to ensure the water isn't too cold.

- **Wear Comfortable Clothing**

When working out, you need to wear something that is super breathable and stretchy. This can help you remain at ease. When you work out, you sweat, so you need to ensure that the clothes you wear are permeable. Not just that, but some moves require you to stretch quite a lot, so you need to ensure that the fabric is suited to stretching.

- **Wear Comfortable Footwear**

You also need to focus on wearing the right shoes. They should be a perfect fit- not too loose or tight. They should have a firm grip on the ground too. This way, you can reduce the risk of falling and can prevent injuries.

- **Warm Up and Cool Down**

Before you start working out, you must warm up first. This helps your body heat up and get ready for the workout. After you are done, you must get your pulse back to normal. For that, you must cool down. Many find warming up and cooling down a sheer waste of time. However, it is extremely crucial. It helps reduce muscle soreness and also reduces the risk of injury quite a lot. Not just that, but it also helps regulate blood flow greatly.

- **Rest**

What is most important is that you listen to your body. No one knows your body better than your own self. So it would be best to focus on what your body is telling you and follow through with it. If you feel like you are getting too tired and your muscles are sore, you need to take a rest day. Remember that exercising is all about making you feel more energetic. The idea is to keep you fit enough to be on the go at all times. So for that, you must focus on having a rest day as needed. This helps you recover and enables you to prepare for the next session too.

- **Take Your Time**

The worst thing that you can do is compare yourself to someone else. Everyone's body is different, meaning everyone has a different way of handling things. Don't beat yourself up if you're taking more time than someone else to get up to a certain level. Remember that we all are different, and it takes time to reach a certain level. Even if you make minimal progress daily, you're on the right track. This is you versus you and not you versus someone else.

Now that you know all about the different forms of workouts, you can choose what works best for you. The idea is to help you get started at the earliest, so that you can age gracefully and take care of your health too. Many diseases can also be prevented if you take precautionary measures and remain physically active.

Importance of Meditation

While physical health is extremely crucial, it is also imperative that you take very good care of your mental health. Meditation is great for older adults. It has substantial effects in terms of calming the mind and body. With so much going on, older adults need to relieve stress, and meditation is ideal for that. It is all about cultivating presence, awareness, and being nonjudgmental.

Benefits of Meditation for Seniors

Here are a few benefits that older people get from meditation, which allows them to boost the quality of their lives.

- **Relieves Stress**

With so much going on in our lives, it is only natural to feel bogged down by stress. Meditation helps you calm down, relieving stress. It enables you to unwind and relax more than anything. Sitting alone and focusing on nothing but your thoughts and the small beauties of life can help you relax. When you meditate, you focus on the negative thoughts, deliberately letting go of all that is bothering you. That allows you to manage your life and all that comes with it.

- **Memory and Retention**

More often than not, older adults tend to struggle with memory and retention. It can be very hard for them to remember things, even things that happened only a few days earlier. Meditation has proven benefits that allow you to focus on things better. These allow you to calm yourself down and channel your inner positivity.

With this, you can also work on strengthening your nervous system. Research has shown that mindful meditation for around thirty minutes a day increases the hippocampus's gray matter, which significantly improves your memory (McGreevy, 2011).

- **Improves Sleep**

Many people have insomnia as they age. They find it harder to sleep at night, even when very tired. Meditation has proven benefits that allow you to sleep better as well. Naturally, when you calm down more, you can sleep much better. Especially those who suffer from chronic illnesses find it even harder to sleep at night. Meditation helps create a very peaceful state of mind, which allows you to calm yourself down and let go of your worries, allowing you to sleep soundly too.

- **Helps Deal with Feelings of Loneliness**

As you age, you see that most people around you are busy with their own lives. This often makes you feel lonely. Meditation helps deal with these feelings as well. When you meditate, you positively channel your inner thoughts, which allows you to be more content. In addition, it allows you to understand yourself in a much better way.

- **Reduces Pain**

Meditation reduces pain in your body, which can result from any chronic illness or diseases associated with age. When you meditate, you allow yourself to calm down, which eventually helps you control your pain too. This is because you meditate on the positive things in life.

- **Helps with Concentration**

As you age, you have so many things you tend to worry about. These act as distractions that don't allow you to focus on the important things in life. Meditation helps you release tension from your body, allowing you to concentrate and increase your attention span. Emotion regulation also becomes possible when you concentrate and try to focus as much as possible.

With so many proven benefits of meditation, you should definitely consider doing it from a young age. Make it a regular part of your routine so that it doesn't seem like something you must take time out for. When you do that, you will see how it positively affects your life.

Misconceptions about Meditation

There are a lot of widespread misconceptions about meditation. Let's clear most of them up:

- There is no specific place that you need to be in to meditate. It can be any place that you like. You need to be at peace there. Not just that, but there should also not be any distractions that prevent you from engaging fully. Try to find a spot that works for you. There is no one-size-fits-all approach here. Try to find out what will suit you best.

- You don't have to let go of all the thoughts in your mind – it's completely impossible for one. Meditation is all about acknowledging your thoughts and feelings and then working your way through them so that you know how to channel your thoughts correctly.

- Many also think that meditation takes up a lot of time. This is not true. You can set aside any time that you have on hand. Even five minutes can work. Once you start, you will see that meditation actually adds time to your day because you will end up being so much more productive. This allows you to work harder.

- There is no specific time to meditate. You can find a time when you are free. Some people like to meditate in the morning, while others like to do it at night since it makes them feel calmer. So it would help to meditate when you think the time is right and when it will calm you down. Remember that you are doing this for yourself, so you need to be the one to find the right time for it.

- Some people also think that meditation is for spiritual or religious people since it is often linked to certain cultural traditions. This is not true. Meditation has nothing to do with your sect or religion. It is solely a mental exercise that allows you to relax, channel your thoughts positively and deal with your worries appropriately.

- Some also think that meditation is only about stress reduction. This is, again, not the case. Meditation has much to do with your physical well-being as well. All you need to do is find a quiet spot. After some time of regular meditation, you will see how it affects your mental and physical health.

Now that you have your doubts clear, you can think of starting meditation. But the question is, how do you start?

How to Meditate?

So first off, you need to find the right spot. It can be any place, even your bedroom. It could be the park near your house, your backyard, or any place you find peaceful and comfortable.

Next, sit on a chair and put your feet up. Remember that the position you sit in needs to be extremely comfortable, so you don't get distracted. It has to be a position that makes the least amount of noise possible. You might have to sit like this for at least fifteen minutes, so try to find the best position.

Thich Nhat Hanh, a master at meditation, said, "Walking meditation unites our body and our mind. We combine our breathing with our steps. When we breathe in, we may take two or three steps. When we breathe out, we may take three, four, or five steps. We pay attention to what is comfortable for our body." Experts recommend meditating for at least fifteen minutes, but what matters most is starting off with what is comfortable for you. Even five to ten minutes can work here.

It would help if you tried to focus as much as possible, so your mind doesn't wander off. Try to be in the moment as much as you can. Try to think of something positive when you find a good spot and a comfortable position. Think about something that makes you happy. It can be a happy moment or a positive emotion. Spell out that positive word in your head. Picture a color that makes you happy, and then try to have that color in your mind for some time. Repeat all of this for as long as you can. You will see how it reduces your stress and makes you feel energized. It will help you see the good in things, thus enabling you to calm down and be happy.

If you are a beginner, there are several meditation podcasts you can also begin with. These will help you focus so much better.

The best part about meditation is that you don't need any equipment. You can start from the comfort of your home, and you will instantly see so many benefits.

Tips to Meditate Effectively

Here are a few meditation tips to help you focus and meditate well.

- **Create a Schedule**

Like all other things, it is natural to become lazy when we don't have a set schedule. So you must make a schedule that can help you calm your thoughts. For example, if the morning works best for you, then maybe you could make a routine, like meditating for ten minutes right after breakfast. Remember that it has to be something that allows you to become more consistent with meditation. This tip is especially very useful for all those who are beginners and are looking to try meditation for the first time.

• Find Others You Can Meditate With

It is recommended that you find a group of people to meditate with if you aren't very comfortable or are generally inconsistent with things. In general, when we start a certain thing with someone, there is some commitment we get bound to. This motivates you to keep going, even when you don't feel like it. In addition, the others you meditate with can help you get back on track whenever you lose motivation.

• Master the Breathwork

It will help if you master the art of breathing in and breathing out first. This is one of the most crucial steps when meditating and can help you meditate in the right way.

• Make Use of Music

Calming music can help you meditate. It can help you calm down and focus on what you are doing. Experts particularly recommend music with meditation for all who are new to it and struggle with anxiety. This is exactly what you need to do if you are looking to start with meditation and remain consistent.

• Get Creative With the Location

Meditating in the same place daily might seem boring after a few days. So to keep your interest levels up, you can experiment with the location. You can try out different places every week, like the park near your house or a place near the river. These can help you feel calmer, allowing you to focus in a much better way as well.

If you aren't too much into starting meditation right away, there are a few mindfulness activities that you can do too. These can allow you to focus on the positive things in life.

Mindfulness Activities

These mindfulness activities will help you see the positive in life, allowing you to focus as much as possible.

- **Spending Time with Nature**

When you spend time with nature, you see so much beauty in God's creation. Being close to nature helps you see the good in life. Imagine sitting by the park near your house and noticing birds chirping; it can help you calm down and unwind. It enables you to observe the beauty of the world that God has created.

- **Journaling**

You can also start off by writing a journal. When you do that, you will see how it helps you focus on all you have to be thankful for, which naturally helps inculcate positive feelings. It also helps boost concentration greatly. This certainly doesn't mean that you have to make it a point to write daily in your journal. It just means that it would be ideal if you started jotting down things you are thankful for. Again, this helps you focus on the good in life, allowing you to make your life so much better.

- **Reading**

Inculcate the habit of reading. Find anything that makes you feel good. It can be an author's work that inspires you. You will see how it helps you improve the quality of your life. You can even read articles about positivity. It will surely have a trickle-down effect on your life too.

- **Set Targeted Goals**

You can set goals about what you wish to achieve. When you do that, you have something productive ahead of you. When you have a target ahead of you, you focus on doing things much better. You channel your energies in the right way too, which is exactly what you need to achieve things in your life.

- **Volunteering**

It is also a great idea to volunteer. You can volunteer anywhere - an orphanage, a hospital, a child care service, anywhere you deem fit. When you help people in need or play your part in doing something positive for society, you will see how much it helps you boost your self-esteem and allows you to look at the good in life. It allows you to see how privileged you are, making you much happier. It makes you understand all God has blessed you with and why you have so much to be thankful for.

- **Appreciate the Small Things**

There is so much good that happens to us every day - a stranger smiling at you, a car giving you space to go first, and so on. You must be very thankful for all these little things since they allow you to see through the good in life. They allow you to fully acknowledge your emotions and understand what all God has given you. Not just that, but appreciating the little things also allows you to make your life so much better since your relationships become stronger.

So the idea is to actively participate in things that make you happy so that you understand the true essence of your life and why you have so much to look forward to and be pleased about.

Importance of Mental Health

Mental health is as important as physical health, but very few people understand this in the modern day and age. Mental health includes our emotional as well as our psychological well-being. It helps determine how we make our life choices and the quality of life that we live too. Whenever we suffer from any physical ailment, we immediately visit the doctor to find out what's wrong. But does the same work for mental health conditions? Unfortunately, it doesn't.

Even when you know and feel something is wrong in your mind, you don't want to get help for it. So generally, our mental health is not very important, which is very unhealthy. We aren't as focused on seeking help when we feel something is wrong, mainly due to the stigma attached to seeking help. We all often face issues when trying to deal with tough situations or when trying to process our emotions. We feel downtrodden, and we feel like our heart is sinking. Yet, the reluctance to get help harms us, making us want to focus less and less on it. The more we choose to ignore it, the greater the harm it does.

This is especially true as we age. Getting older in itself can be a mental challenge. When we see our health deteriorating, and when we understand that we are nearing the age where it's time to go finally, we find it hard to deal with it. We find it hard to cope with the fact that this is a regular life cycle. Feelings of loneliness are also very common when you're young, which can take a major toll on your quality of life.

So it would help if you focused as much as possible on your mental health since it is a central part of your overall being. It affects your self-esteem and also affects the way that you handle different challenges in life. Not only is your mental health important for your own self, but it also allows you to get through your life by building your relationships with others. Research has shown that around 15% of adults over the age of 60 suffer from various mental disorders. This statistic shows that it is high time we learn how to deal with mental health issues to focus on the quality of our lives and build a better life for ourselves.

Mental Health Issues that Older Adults Face

So what are some mental health issues that older adults face? Here are a few of the main ones.

- **Depression**

Depression is one of the most common mental health issues in older adults. When they see that they are at the stage of life where things only go downhill, feelings of lasting sadness set in, which tend to affect the overall quality of their life too. Most people who feel tired, have trouble sleeping, or are just grumpy and irritable show signs of depression too. Primary caregivers can ask certain questions and diagnose depression in older adults.

- **Anxiety**

Anxiety is also prevalent in older adults. The feeling of nervousness and impatience to know what's coming next can make them feel agitated. Constant worrying is also one of the major reasons that older people suffer from anxiety. In addition, the constant fear about things like financial issues, dependence on others, and feelings of being left alone eventually lead to anxiety. Alcohol and substance abuse are also the main reasons why anxiety persists in older adults.

- **Bipolar Disorder**

Do you often see older adults having unusual shifts in their mood? They might feel very happy at one given point, and at another, they might feel very down. Chances are that they have bipolar disorder. This disorder can become very severe and cause many further issues if left unchecked. This can also lead to other problems, including sleeping, racing thoughts, and processing information. The thing with bipolar disorder is that it is often confused with dementia or other cognitive issues. But the sooner it is diagnosed, the better it is because the chances of managing it are much higher.

- **Dementia**

Dementia is also one of the most common mental health issues people face as they age. However, it isn't a normal part of aging. There are several forms that dementia can take, and one of them is Alzheimer's. In dementia, the normal brain cells stop working, impairing cognitive function and not allowing retaining things. As a result of dementia, people may face memory loss, understanding problems, poor judgment, and problems with reading and writing. While the exact cause of dementia in older adults isn't known, people must recognize that there is a problem and help those suffering from it get help.

- **Obsessive Compulsive Disorder**

Obsessive-compulsive disorder is a very common issue in the elderly. It involves uncontrollable thoughts and unnecessary compulsions. This disorder can interfere with a person's day-to-day affairs and also cause a hindrance in the way that they think. Examples include washing hands repeatedly and checking the same place repeatedly to see if something is still there.

These are the most common mental health issues that older adults face. Therefore, you must get help for them if you see them suffering from any of these. The following section will help you understand the vital signs that can help you know if they are facing specific mental health issues.

Signs of Mental Health Issues in the Elderly

Now that you know the common mental health issues with older people, it is essential to look at signs that point out mental health issues. Family members can only help seniors get help when they understand them. So here are a few signs that can tell you that something is going wrong in their minds and that they are in need of help.

- **Social Isolation**

If you see the elderly isolating themselves and preferring to stay alone over anything else, chances are they are struggling to deal with something happening in their head. They might not be able to talk about it most time. The hesitance can come from a fear of not being able to make the other person understand what is bothering them. It can also come from the fear of being judged by others. So the best solution is to avoid others and try to deal with their problems themselves. What this eventually does is that it makes their mental health even, disallowing them from living a quality life.

- **Confusion**

Often, the elderly struggle to make sense of what is happening around them. They might seem confused and might not be fully able to comprehend things. This is why they also struggle when trying to make decisions in life. This is also a sign of some chemical imbalance in their heads that can tell you something is wrong inside and that they are trying to deal with things but struggling. Confusion and disorientation are also early signs of dementia in the elderly.

- **Appetite Changes**

If you see that the older adults around you are overeating all of a sudden or not eating at all, then chances are that something is going wrong and that they aren't mentally stable. It can hint at any underlying mental health issue, so they need to be checked for it and surely need medical help.

- **Sleep Changes**

The importance of sleep is something that cannot be undermined. This is especially true when you age. This book covers an entire chapter on the importance of ample sleep. The idea here is to point out how changes in sleep patterns, like not being able to sleep or sleeping too much, can also hint toward mental health issues. It may be a sign of some significant mental disorder.

- **Feelings of Hopelessness**

Suppose you see that the elderly people around you seem too hopeless and unwilling to do things that once interested them greatly. In that case, chances are that they are losing interest due to some underlying mental health condition. It is quite common for older adults to lose hope as they age. They might feel like they aren't good enough and that nothing is left in their lives to look forward to. This can make them feel very paranoid too.

- **Suicidal Thoughts**

Suicidal thoughts are very common in older adults. When they struggle to find meaning in their lives or don't see anything worth living for, suicidal thoughts may come into their minds, affecting how they live. These thoughts can also be perilous. Suicidal thoughts are one of the main signs that can tell you that there is something wrong in their heads and that they need help. One of the main reasons that suicidal thoughts come to their mind is because they feel lonely and don't see any reason to continue living. Other reasons include loss of self-sufficiency, chronic illnesses, grief over losing loved ones, and financial problems.

- **Changes in Personal Hygiene**

Sometimes, you may even see that older adults might not find the energy to bathe or brush their teeth. They may start finding tasks like these mundane and might not end up doing these at all. This is a sign that they are suffering from specific mental health issues that are really bothering them, disallowing them from functioning correctly.

- **Memory Loss**

It is very common to see older adults who can't remember things. It is a sign that tells you something is wrong inside, leading them to forget things. This is also a sign that they are suffering from one problem or the other and that their mental health condition isn't stable enough.

If you see any of these signs in your loved ones, then it is high time you understand that they need help, and you get a consultation done with a mental health practitioner who can help diagnose any such issues.

Getting Help

If you see these mental health issues becoming more prevalent, you must get help. However, getting professional help for these mental health issues is something that is seen as taboo. For that, it is important that there is greater awareness about mental health issues and why they pose a huge risk to your life.

Apart from getting professional help, here are a few tips that can help you stay mentally healthy and improve your quality of life significantly.

- **Stay Connected with Family and Loved Ones**

More often, feelings of loneliness set in as you grow older. These feelings can make you sink and sad without having anything to look forward to. So to avoid these feelings, you must always stay connected with your loved ones. Try to spend time with those you love. That will help you look at the good in life and will also help you see how there are so many people who love you. If you live away from your loved ones, you can easily stay in touch with them using technology. This will allow you to remain connected and make you feel a much better place mentally.

- **Remain Busy**

Having too much time on hand and nothing to do can make your thoughts wander off to unneeded places. This can make you feel useless. It can make you feel like you have nothing to do. It can make you feel like you aren't adding value to anything happening around you. So it would help if you try to remain as busy as possible. What you remain busy doing is entirely up to you.

You could pick a hobby that is productive and allows you to keep mentally stimulated as well. You could also keep yourself busy doing something productive like teaching or volunteering. What you do doesn't matter as long as it is something you like and as long as it keeps you mentally stimulated. This will help you see the good in life. Not just that, but when you see purpose in what you do, you will surely see life as worthwhile and will not find your thoughts wandering off to other places. Again, when you invest your time in something you don't like, it won't be of any help. This will help you see the good in life. So, one should spend their time wisely to stay busy.

- **Participate in House Chores**

Usually, older people are seen to spend time mostly sleeping or doing something that isn't really adding value. Instead, you are highly recommended to participate in household chores like washing dishes or cooking and cleaning. When you do that, you will feel very useful and find yourself helping your loved ones do something they would otherwise have to do without help. So when you participate in household chores, you will see how productive it helps you feel. Not just that, but you will also find yourself very busy doing something that is actually of use. It also helps fulfill the purpose of helping you stay connected with your loved ones.

- **Stay Mentally Stimulated**

Whatever you do, you must make sure that you are putting your mind to some use. It can be anything that stimulates you and allows you to think about things. For example, reading, writing, learning a new language or playing an instrument. All of these come as part of you doing something very productive. This practice can allow you to put yourself to some use, which means that you can see the good in life when you do so. In addition, it will allow you to put your brain to doing something great, which will eventually prove very healthy for your brain. However, when you leave things aside, one day or later, you will start feeling lousy and irritated with everything else.

- **Volunteer**

When you do something that satisfies you, you will see how much it will help you see the good in life. When you help others, the satisfaction that comes with it is unmatched. Volunteering is one of those things that help you work for a cause and allows you to see how you can positively contribute to building a better society. So, it would help if you always were focused on doing something that helps you remain content with yourself. It can be anything like volunteering at an old age home where you can connect with the elderly or at a child care center. Volunteering also helps you stay grounded and see the good in things.

Keep a Pet

Often, old people don't have anyone to spend time with, which inculcates greater feelings of loneliness. They crave companionship, but sometimes they don't have an option. Either they don't have any family, or they live far away. The best thing to do in such a case is to have a pet. Being a pet parent can allow you to feel very loved. It is a full-time job, so you will find yourself mostly always busy caring for the pet. You can buy any pet you like, and then you can care for the pet like your own child. You will see how it helps you remain occupied doing something highly productive.

- **Stay Positive**

You must always try to remain positive, no matter the situation. Always try to focus on the good things in life. That being said, it is surely easier said than done. With so much going on around you, you might find it hard to focus on the good that is happening. But it would help if you make a conscious effort to do so.

- **Practice Gratitude**

I once read, "If you concentrate on finding whatever is good in every situation, you will discover that your life will suddenly be filled with gratitude, a feeling that nurtures the soul." This has stuck with me ever since. Gratitude is great for your soul since it allows you to see the good in things. It allows you to focus on the good things in your life, which is exactly what you need to live a much better life. So try to make thankfulness more of an approach for yourself. That way, you will be able to focus on all that you have. It will show you how privileged you are to have many blessings. It will make you understand life better, giving you a greater perspective. So you must always try to focus on this since it will allow you to have your things sorted much better.

- **Relax**

Try to practice some relaxation techniques. When you do that, you will see how it helps you calm yourself down. We have to deal with so many things in our lives daily. You can't shut your mind entirely and try to block everything. Even when we try harder to ignore ongoing things in our minds, something always grabs our attention. So, what you can do is find a coping mechanism that allows you to look at things a certain way. That will allow you to focus better and will also allow you to understand things properly.

Hence one should try to do things that make them feel relaxed. This can be anything at all. For example, you can try to meditate, even go out for a walk in the park, or talk to a loved one. Anything that makes you feel calmer and allows you to block all negative thoughts for a while will surely help you unwind and will help you see the good in things. There is no hard and fast rule about what you should be doing. It depends entirely on what helps you calm down.

Getting Help

Several people suffer from mental health issues; therefore, it should be given utmost importance. If you ever feel like you aren't doing well mentally, it is up to you to seek help. Always tell yourself that your health matters and that there is no shame in asking for help. In the same way, you should consult a doctor when facing any issues with your physical health, and you must also visit a mental health practitioner when you feel things aren't in your hands or that you're suffering mentally. I repeat, there is no shame in talking about mental health-related issues. Instead, when you seek help, it creates awareness for others as well.

Now, another question arises, who do you seek help from? If someone is suicidal, you can call 911 for help since it is an emergency. But if it isn't an emergency, you can seek help from a regular doctor, who will walk you through how you're feeling and will make you identify symptoms first. Then, if they feel like you're doing alright physically, they will refer you to a mental health professional, who will then diagnose what exactly is wrong.

Healthcare Professionals:

Many healthcare professionals can help you deal with this:

- *General Practitioner*: A general practitioner is someone who deals with a variety of health issues. They will do a full checkup to see what is wrong with you first. Next, they will identify underlying causes and will check for symptoms. These doctors are known to treat a wide variety of medical conditions and can also check you up and help you.

- *Physician Assistant*: These aren't trained doctors, but they can help you identify certain symptoms. Under a doctor's supervision, they can help treat several mental disorders.

- *Psychiatrists*: These are medical doctors highly specialized in dealing with different types of mental illnesses. They can also prescribe medications after fully understanding your mental health condition. These doctors are highly trained and have dealt with various cases, so you won't have to worry.

- *Psychologist*: These aren't medical doctors but have very advanced degrees in psychology. They are trained in dealing with patients who are suffering from one or the other form of mental illness. They usually engage in talk therapy after talking to patients and trying to understand what they are going through. They then provide counseling and allow patients to explore different ways in which they can solve their issues. They aren't trained to provide medication for different mental health issues, but they can diagnose the problem and help deal with it better through counseling sessions.

So you can go to any of these people, depending on the kind of treatment that you are looking for. But there is one thing that you should remember; you should never shy away from getting help. Your mental health condition is directly related to the quality of your life, so it should always be a priority for you.

No matter what someone tells you, you must focus on ensuring that your mental health comes first. When you do that, you will see how great your life becomes. This is one of the most important factors affecting healthy aging; hence, you should always be mindful.

The Art of the Hobby

At an older age, you have generally crossed the busy age of your life and have much time at hand. Many older people get extremely bored when they don't have much to do. This gives way to idle thoughts, which aren't always very positive. It is highly recommended that you keep yourself as busy as possible to immerse yourself in positive thoughts, focusing on the good in life. Otherwise, you will not be able to live a peaceful life since idleness comes with various negative factors.

Benefits of Hobbies for Seniors

For older people, it is ideal to have some hobbies that keep you busy. Here are a few benefits of hobbies.

- **Stress Relief**

Hobbies allow you to release stress and feel much calmer. With hobbies, you can keep yourself busy doing something you like, so your mind won't wander off to other places. Hobbies allow you to take some time out for yourself and calm down. You can let go of your negative emotions when you inculcate hobbies.

- **Sense of Purpose**

Hobbies give you a sense of purpose, meaning you have something to look forward to. When you engage in something positive, your mind surely functions in a better way. When there is a goal ahead of you, you can work your way up to it and have something that keeps you busy. So as important as it is to be busy, it is also important to do something positive.

- **Sense of Accomplishment**

When you accomplish something positive, you naturally feel great about yourself, knowing that you have done something great.

Try to achieve something challenging, and put your utmost effort into accomplishing your goal. Once accomplished, you will feel the best version of yourself.

- **Hidden Talents**

Many times, you don't even know what talents you have. Hobbies help you explore these talents, allowing you to become so much better at things. It is a great path to self-discovery that allows you to understand yourself much better.

- **Physical Health**

Some hobbies also allow you to become much stronger. For example, taking up a hobby like swimming or hiking can help you make yourself much fitter physically. Hobbies like these are ones that you should have to keep yourself entertained and work on making yourself stronger. Older adults are often restricted to swimming and hiking; they can consider walking as their hobby, which will help them stay fit for several years.

Hobby Ideas for Older Adults

Here are a few hobby ideas that can help you stay busy.

- **Reading**

Reading is a great hobby to have. Not only does it keeps you busy, but it also makes you extremely knowledgeable. Reading is known to help with improving memory. Not just that, but it also helps your brain become much sharper, which eventually also makes your decision-making skills much better. Apart from that, it also helps you reduce stress levels. When you immerse yourself in an interesting story, you forget about your worries, and hence can reduce your stress levels. For those who struggle with sleep, reading can help you sleep well too. You can read your favorite book right before bedtime and will slowly notice how it helps you sleep much better.

- **Gardening**

Gardening is also one of the best hobbies you can have. For those who love nature, it is a great way to stay busy and focused on the good things in life. It can be extremely fulfilling to sow some seeds and watch plants grow; it gives you undefinable peace. A study done in 2015 showed that two fifty-minute pot-planting sessions help improve stamina (Graaf, 2016). Not just that, but it also helps the brain function. It isn't hard to see why so many people absolutely love gardening. It helps them remain busy doing something highly fulfilling and productive.

- **Writing**

Writing is yet another great hobby to have. When you jot your thoughts down, it helps you organize yourself much better. Not just that, it also helps you understand yourself in terms of being organized with your thoughts. It can also be extremely entertaining to write, especially if you are a fiction lover. You can let your thoughts go wild. It can be more fun than you can ever imagine. Especially when you write on a topic you are passionate about, you will see how much it helps you. More than anything, it helps stimulate your brain and keeps your mind sharp. It also helps with eye coordination skills. For those with a creative side, writing can be a game-changer. It can be your creative outlet, allowing you to put your skills to the best use. Also, writing helps you when no one is listening to you. For example, if you feel lonely or distant from your loved ones, you can easily write down your thoughts or feelings on a piece of paper, and thus it can give you a feeling of relief.

- **Cooking**

Cooking is also one of the best hobbies to have. It keeps you distracted and also helps you feel fulfilled. You can stay busy by cooking meals for yourself and your loved ones. The feeling of giving joy to your loved ones by feeding them something you made yourself can make you feel highly accomplished. Those who cook often know that it helps you keep yourself occupied doing something healthy. You can create different meal plans and experiment with many recipes online. Not only is this very exciting, but it can also help you become the master of a very essential life skill.

- **Bird Watching**

If you are a nature lover, watching birds can be very exciting. It is a great way to relax and admire God's creations. It helps the elderly fight off stress by indulging in something good for their mental health. It is also known to help with age-related cognitive decline.

- **Traveling**

Nothing can be more exciting than traveling the world and seeing different locations. Traveling offers fascinating opportunities to learn and grow. It is also one of the best ways to keep you as entertained as possible. It can be rewarding in many ways. You can pick out your top holiday spots and can go out exploring with your spouse or your loved ones. You will see how much that helps you relax and unwind. It also helps you stay physically fit.

- **Volunteering**

Volunteering for any cause can be extremely fulfilling. Not only can it help you stay busy doing something productive, but it will also help you feel great about yourself. When you give back to society, it gives you a feeling of self-satisfaction that is unmatched. Volunteering doesn't mean investing in the greater good. You can volunteer at any place that you like. It will help you see how you are blessed and that there are many people in dire need of help. It will also give you a feeling of self-fulfillment to do your part to make this world a much better place.

• Solving Puzzles

If you are one to enjoy doing creative things that stimulate your brain, then solving puzzles is a great idea. It can be exciting and very satisfying. In addition, you can solve different types of puzzles. This can help you remain busy. You can do jigsaw puzzles, word games, and other mobile application games. It increases your brain activity and thus provides you an easy escape to stay away from all the worries and stress.

• Dancing

If you enjoy staying active and are a music lover, you should try creating a dancing routine. It can help you stay active and in shape too. Dancing is basically an exercise without making you feel like you are exercising. So it helps fulfill the purpose of keeping you fit and entertaining. You can even join a dance school or have a dance instructor who guides you every step of the way. If you have someone in the house who shares the same interest, you can ask them to be your dance partner. It can make your dancing sessions all the more interesting.

• Fishing

If you live by the water, fishing is a great idea. Being by the water is very relaxing on its own. Fishing can be an interesting pastime to help you make the most of your time. It can also make you feel highly productive. There are several different fishing techniques that you can learn, too. If you want to take up fishing professionally, you can buy fishing gear to help you up your game.

• Painting

Painting is also one of the best hobbies if you like playing with colors. It allows you to explore your creative side and work on anything you like. All you need is some colors and some painting canvas. Then you can unleash your creativity and paint what you like. It can be anything that inspires you. You can paint sunsets, scenery, wildlife, and anything you find interesting – the sky is the limit.

- **Adopting a Pet**

One of the things that can keep you most occupied is adopting a pet. It helps you keep the feeling of loneliness away. You become a parent to your fur baby, as they add so much love and light to your life. When you have a pet to take care of, you don't need anyone near you as they fill your life with neverending happiness. Being a pet parent is a full-time job. It means you have to take care of what your pet eats, take them out on a walk, entertain them, schedule visits to the vet, and so on. So if you're an animal lover, there can be nothing better than adopting a pet.

- **Playing Board Games**

For those who like to explore their creative side and play games, it is a great idea to play board games. With so many different options available, you can choose the one that seems the most challenging. Board games like scrabble help you stay focused and stimulate your mind. They also sharpen your thinking skills, allowing you to reduce the risk of cognitive decline. It is always best to keep yourself busy doing something productive in which you have to stimulate your brain.

- **Joining Community Groups**

A lot of older people feel a lack of connection. They feel very lonely, so joining community groups is a great idea. When you do that, you can interact with like-minded people, which can help you stay as connected as possible. It helps you understand things in a much better way and also allows you to get useful advice from all who are at the same stage of their life as you. This can help you remain extremely entertained regarding what other people your age like to indulge in. It can also help you stay up to date with what is happening around you. It is always nice to have wonderful people around whom you can speak to. In community groups, people are often seen doing things together, like yoga, singing, etc. So, it depends entirely on what you want.

- **Crafting**

If you have a creative side, you can try crafting. Clay-making, quilting, and knitting are all extremely interesting things to do. They are therapeutic for some seniors as well. They help you unwind and give you a sense of achievement, knowing that you have done something extremely productive. To see your vision come to life can be extremely satisfying. This is also a great hobby idea for those who like to use their hands to do things. You can find different clay-making ideas on the internet and start making them after you buy all the materials you need.

- **Teaching**

As a senior, you have a lot of life experience. You can easily share this with others around you. Sharing life lessons and experiences can help so many others around you, who would then be able to live their life much better. Your experiences can help others shape their lives and make the quality of their lives much better. You can also start teaching professionally if you have specialized in a particular area. It can be any subject that you are an expert at. Imparting knowledge is one of the things that can help you feel good about yourself. Not only that, but it can also be extremely enjoyable for you. It also helps you generate some extra cash, and who doesn't like that, right?

Sleep and Healthy Aging

Getting ample sleep is essential for all age groups. But as you age, it becomes even more critical. Your body needs to be well-rested to function at full capacity. A good night's sleep allows you to improve your concentration and memory. Not just that, but it also allows you to boost your immune system, hence preventing diseases. Older adults who don't get adequate sleep are more likely to suffer from depression, fatigue, diabetes, weight problems, and many other health issues. So you need to ensure that you make your sleep a priority. Your body needs a certain amount of rest. Without that, you will surely see hampered productivity.

Most older people notice changes in their sleep patterns as they age. They might find it harder to sleep at night and nap during the day. Not just that, they might also find themselves unable to keep up with their sleep routines. Before we get to healthy sleeping tips, you must understand that aging does affect your sleep. Changes in the body's internal clock cause this to happen. We have a master clock in our brain called the hypothalamus. This has around 20,000 cells and is what forms the suprachiasmatic nucleus. Changes in sleeping patterns are usually seen due to suprachiasmatic nucleus aging.

Besides that, mental and physical health conditions are also major factors that affect your sleep cycles. Those suffering from chronic illnesses are more likely to have poor-quality sleep. Not just that, but they are also usually seen to get less than six hours of sleep a night. Another major cause of sleep problems can be medications. Most older people have multiple health issues for which they consume certain medications. Those medications can have side effects and can also hamper your sleep. For example, anti-depressants are known to cause insomnia.

Another factor that affects sleep in older adults is lifestyle. When you age, you spend lesser time doing productive things. For example, if you retire, you might spend more time at home. This might even mean that you spend more time napping during the day, which is why you can't seem to fall asleep at night. In addition, if you suffer from stress and anxiety, then that might also lead to sleep issues.

A common misconception is that older people need lesser sleep. This is far from being true. Very often, people ask how much sleep older adults need. The truth is that everyone has different bodily requirements. However, most healthy adults require seven to nine hours of sleep each night to function well. If you feel rested during the day and don't tire out when doing regular activities, this is a sign that you are getting enough sleep.

Furthermore, mostly older adults need about the same amount of sleep as all adults – 7 to 9 hours each night. But, older people tend to go to sleep earlier and get up earlier than they did when they were younger.

Common Sleep Issues in Older Adults

Most older adults suffer from chronic sleep issues. These affect the quality of their lives and also affect their daily activities. Here are a few common sleep issues that older people face:

- **Pain**

Many people feel constant pain in several parts of their bodies. This can be a result of any chronic illness or an age factor. Regardless, it interferes with their sleep patterns, disallowing them from getting enough sleep in a day. Some might even wake up several times in the night due to pain and discomfort.

- **Sleep Apnea**

Sleep apnea is a problem that leads to disruptions when trying to sleep due to oxygen not reaching the brain. Sometimes, the upper airway in the body gets blocked, which means that people can't breathe well when sleeping. This causes huge issues for them. This problem affects around 20 to 60% of people over 65. More often than not, this problem starts with snoring and then becomes more problematic over time.

- **Restless Leg Syndrome**

Sometimes, older adults find it hard to remain still when sleeping. They keep moving their legs during sleep, affecting their sleep. It affects those for whom these leg-moving episodes last longer.

- **Frequent Urination**

As you grow older, your bladder becomes weaker. This means that the urge to urinate becomes much more frequent. You might find it hard to hold it in, even at night. So the need to urinate frequently affects your sleep routine, and you might have to wake up very often.

- **Insomnia**

Insomnia is one of the most frequent sleep issues many people face as they age. Changes in routine and regular medication might affect the way you fall asleep. So you might find it hard to go to bed every night. However, it is possible to deal with this issue with regular treatment and medication.

These are usually all the issues that are related to sleep. Therefore, you must focus as much as you can on improving your sleep patterns. This way, you can save yourself from these problems as much as possible.

Diagnosing Sleep Disorders

If you are facing sleep issues, you must visit the doctor to get these issues diagnosed.

So, how are sleep disorders diagnosed?

Your doctor will ask you a few questions related to your sleep patterns. They will also conduct a detailed analysis of your sleep problems and any other underlying conditions that may cause this. Suppose you persistently suffer from sleep issues and find yourself unable to concentrate during the daytime. In that case, chances are that you are suffering from serious sleep issues that need to be cured.

If your doctor suspects you are suffering from serious sleep issues, they can get polysomnography done. They might even conduct an at-home sleep test. This will help them understand if you are facing any issues. In a sleep study, the technician monitors your body movements, breathing patterns, snoring noises, heart rate, and brain activity. By monitoring all of this, they can tell whether or not you suffer from any serious sleep issues and how you can deal well with these problems.

Next, you must know how you can sleep well.

Tips for A Good Night's Sleep

Here are a few tips that can help you sleep well.

- **Stick to a Sleep Schedule**

The first and most important thing is to make a sleep schedule for yourself. You must target at least eight hours of sleep a night. Then, try to adjust your schedule around it. This may seem hard, especially if you are retired and don't have much to do during the day. But you need to understand how important a good night's sleep is. It allows you to rest well and will also allow you to function properly. Go to bed at the same time each day and wake up at a specific time in the morning. Initially, setting a very tight schedule for yourself might seem hard. But try to make a conscious effort to act upon this, and you will see how things work out for you. You will see how much it helps you, making you much more productive in the day.

- **Do Something Relaxing Before You Sleep**

If you find it hard to put yourself to sleep at night, try to do something relaxing before you go to bed. There are no hard and fast rules about what you should be doing, as long as it helps you get relaxed. For example, maybe you could read something that helps you feel great. You could even take a nice hot shower or lie in bed and speak to someone you love. When you do this, you will automatically feel yourself much at ease, which will allow you to relax and will allow you to sleep well too. When your mind is at ease, it will be much easier to shut it off before you sleep.

- **Create a Peaceful Environment**

When going to bed, try to create a very restful environment; turn the lights off and keep your room cool. Ensure that there is no notice. Try to put all your electronic gadgets in silent mode so they don't disrupt your sleep. Try to avoid the use of screens right before you sleep. When you create a peaceful and restful environment, you will notice how much easier it is to fall asleep. Do anything that creates a very peaceful environment, allowing you to sleep well.

- **Don't Consume Caffeine Late at Night**

In the latter part of the day, try to limit caffeine intake. While it has numerous health benefits, it can also keep you up since it boosts energy levels and enhances focus levels. It also stimulates brain activity. So when you near your bedtime, try to limit your use of caffeine so that you can sleep well and shut your brain off entirely. If you crave a cup of coffee, try to have decaffeinated coffee. That will surely help you a lot.

- **Reduce Day Time Naps**

If you have a habit of sleeping during the day, try to reduce it. Some people who have developed this habit over the years or those who get very tired during the day might find this very hard. But it would help if you cut back on this slowly and gradually. When you do this, you will see that you will naturally find it very easy to go to sleep at night. However, you will surely get more tired during the day, and your body will need that rest at night. If you have to sleep during the day, try limiting the time. You could get a power nap of thirty minutes or less- just enough to help you feel rested.

- **Limit Alcohol Intake**

Try to limit your intake of alcohol. Alcohol affects your sleep hormones and increases your sleep apnea symptoms and snoring. So try to keep that at a minimum. Alcohol is also known to alter melatonin production at night. For someone who is used to having a lot of alcohol during the day, this can be problematic to a very great extent. So try to take a step at a time and reduce your intake as much as possible to sleep well at night.

- **Exercise Regularly**

One of the numerous benefits of exercising is that it allows you to sleep well. When you exercise, you tire yourself out during the day, which eventually improves the quality of your sleep as well. Don't expect this to happen overnight. When you get into the habit of exercising regularly, you will see how it helps over time. When you exercise, your body exerts itself, which allows you to go to bed peacefully.

- **Eat Smartly**

Nutrition also plays a huge role in your sleeping patterns. Try to focus on having a healthy diet where you eat from all food groups. Try to cut back on all sugary foods and refined carbs. These can trigger wakefulness at night and disrupt your sleeping patterns. Another helpful tip is to avoid having a big meal at night. When you feel too heavy, it might not allow you to sleep well, either. So, try to limit yourself from overeating at night. Take your big meals during the day, if necessary, and eat very light meals at night.

- **Reduce Stress Levels**

If something is bothering you, it can keep you up at night. You might find yourself staying up, worrying about things happening in your life. The focus must surely be on managing your worries. Try to deal with your problems in the best way. You could try different stress management techniques to see which works for you. Stress affects our lives in unimaginable ways. Even if we try to control all that is bothering us, it seldom works in our favor. You might subconsciously be awake, worrying about different things in your life. So, keep trying different techniques until they work out for you.

If you have tried most things but still find it hard to sleep at night, you should visit a doctor for a detailed examination. The doctor will guide you through the process and check you well to see the issue.

Skin Health and Aging

As you grow older, your skin ages too. You might see your skin becoming more fragile over time. Not just that, but you might even notice wrinkles much earlier on. Why does that happen? As you grow older, your skin becomes thinner due to losing fat. Due to that reason, it does not look as smooth and plump as it once did. This tends to take a toll on your self-esteem as well. You no longer find yourself being comfortable in your skin.

First, I want to point out that your outward appearance does not define you. Many people do not accept that they are aging, and when they see their skin getting fragile, they become very conscious. It is important to train our minds to accept the reality of aging. All phases of our lives are equally beautiful, and we must fully embrace them. Try to understand that aging is a natural process, and you cannot expect things to remain the same your entire life. When you age, you experience things differently, and your body changes too. It would help if you never let anything take a toll on your mental health. What you can do is work towards building a healthier you!

Several factors affect the way your skin looks. These include your lifestyle, diet, genetic factors, and personal habits. For example, if you tend to eat unhealthy foods, that will surely show up on your skin, increasing your acne. Furthermore, if you are a smoker, you will see premature skin wrinkles.

Skin Changes with Age

Here are a few common skin changes that you can see as you age:

- Rougher skin

- Bruises on the skin

- Wrinkles

- Transparent skin

- Loosely hanging skin

- Fragile skin

If you see any of these on your skin, you must understand that all of this is very common and that you will see them more often than not as you age. It would help if you were one to understand how to deal well with it. More than anything, you need to inculcate healthy habits. These habits allow you to have more youthful-looking skin.

The sun also affects your skin in many ways. Direct exposure to sunlight for elongated periods damages fibers in your skin called elastin. This causes the skin to sag. It also becomes weaker, making your skin more prone to bruises. While the skin does repair itself, there is nothing you can do to stop sun damage. Only protective measures you take over time can help you build healthier skin.

Skin Care Tips for Healthy Aging

Here are a few skincare tips to help you have more youthful-looking skin. Jessica Wu, a dermatologist, says, "Your skin is a living organ that changes over time. Adjusting your skincare to accommodate these changes will help your skin stay healthy and looking its best."

- **Protect Your Skin From the Sun**

Direct exposure to sunlight can affect your skin in unimaginable ways. So it would be best if you tried to protect it at all times. It is very hard for those working outside to avoid sun exposure. So what do you do then? First, you must use sunscreen with an SPF of at least 15. Apply it generously on your face every day before you step out of the house. This will help protect your skin from the harmful rays of the sun. If you have to remain in the sun for some hours at a stretch, try reapplying for it whenever you need to. Try to seek shade if you can when the sun shines bright. This will help protect your skin from massive damage. It is also recommended that you wear clothing that protects your skin. Long-sleeved shirts and long pants are a great idea to help you stay protected from the sun. If possible, also wear a hat.

- **Keep Your Skin Clean**

The most important thing you can do for your skin is to keep it as clean as possible. Never allow dirt to settle on your face. Dirt and other contaminants can cause your skin to break out. So whenever you come home from the outside, wash your skin with the face wash that suits you or your dermatologist recommended. This will allow your skin to look fresher and help keep dirt off. One of the most common mistakes many people make is washing their face with hot water. Extremely hot water rids your face with natural oils. So it would be best if you try to keep it as lukewarm as possible. Similarly, you must also try to avoid extra cold water. Unfortunately, that doesn't allow you to eliminate all the excess dirt.

- **Moisturize Your Skin**

After you wash your skin, you must moisturize it. This allows your skin to retain moisture and not get extra dry and flaky. Massage the moisturizer slowly onto your skin, gently moving upwards as needed. You will notice how fresh your skin looks. This step is especially very important for all those who have dry skin. Water will make your skin dry up even more. So after every wash, you must ensure that you moisturize it.

- **Be Gentle With Your Skin**

Don't use any harsh products on your skin. Products with extra chemicals only end up harming your skin in the long run. So use all mild products. For example, while it is very important to use facial cleansers, ensure that you use mild ones. If you use harsh ones, they will end up irritating your skin. You might then notice your skin breaking out very often. So try to keep such products away. Some people also believe in rigorous exfoliation. While exfoliation is great for your skin since it allows all the extra dirt to get washed away, extra exfoliation will only end up damaging your skin and might even make it weaker.

- **Know Your Skin**

Understand your skin, and know your skin type. Once you do that, you can only use the right products for your skin. The products that might work for you might not work for someone else. So try to understand your skin type, and then do your research to find the right skin products. More often than not, we use products that others recommend without understanding if they are good for our skin. So first, research and then use products that work for you.

- **Use Makeup Wisely**

Some people wear makeup every day. While it is a personal choice, you must try to limit your use of makeup. That will allow your skin to breathe and stay in its natural element. On days you choose to take off, maybe you could have makeup-free days. You will see how your skin feels so much healthier when you do that. Another very important factor you need to consider is the cleanliness of your makeup tools. Always keep your makeup brushes very clean. You have no idea how many germs they could be carrying. They are breeding grounds for bacteria and dead skin cells. Beauty experts recommend that you clean your brushes every week. That allows you to eliminate any extra germs they might be carrying.

- **Use Face Masks**

Face masks can do magic for your skin. Make masking a regular part of your skincare routine. There are so many face masks that you can buy over the counter. So try to find something that works for you and stick to it. There are so many DIY face masks that so many people swear by. Most of these use honey, lemon, and baking soda, amongst other ingredients. If you are not getting anything in particular, wash your face with a mixture of gram flour and milk; it will refresh your skin like no other. So you can research and try to see which one works for you. One thing is sure: you must never miss out on your skincare routine. It is very normal to laze out and then forget about it altogether. Remember that when you take care of your skin and make it a priority, it shows up on the skin, which remains fresh in your later life.

- **Use Retinoids**

As you age, your skin might lose collagen. This is the protein that allows the skin to look smooth and lifted. You might notice your skin looking much more creased when you lose collagen. To make up for that, you can use retinoids. Essentially, retinoids are prescription versions of vitamin A that allow your skin to feel fresh and look younger for the most part. There are many retinoid creams that you can find over the counter. Try to use those to help you remain to look fresh as ever.

- **Use Vitamin C**

Vitamin C is one of the best topical ingredients for glowing skin. You can use this regardless of your skin type. It promotes balanced pigmentation and allows your skin tone to become much brighter. It also allows for greater elastic production in your body. So try to find products that have vitamin C in them.

- **Exfoliate Weekly**

Try to exfoliate regularly. When you do that, your dead skin cells will shed off and leave your skin feeling much fresher. You can use any scrub that suits your skin, but you need to be sure that it does not irritate your skin. Try to use a scrub that is gentle on your skin. Scrubs with round particles are highly recommended since they aren't very harsh on the skin.

- **Don't Pick Your Skin**

What was the last time you touched your face and picked a pimple? Let's admit it; we aren't very careful with this. We tend to touch our skin very often, which causes massive damage. Generally, your hands possess many germs. So, consciously or subconsciously, try to keep your hands off your face. When you do that, you will see how great you feel. When you pick your skin, you give way to bacteria entering the skin and making any underlying skin condition worse. You also allow your skin to break out more, causing all the more issues.

- **Have a Balanced Diet**

You must ensure that you eat well for everything related to your health. Try to include many fruits, vegetables, whole grains, and lean proteins in your diet to have more youthful-looking skin. People at young age avoid eating healthily, and thus they face numerous deficiencies in their later lives. In contrast, when you eat healthily, it shows up on your skin because your skin gets all the necessary nutrients that it needs. Also, you must drink plenty of water every day. At least eight to ten glasses a day is a must to keep your skin hydrated and ensure that it looks very healthy. You must try to reduce extra sugar, which affects your skin adversely and allows for premature aging.

- **Don't Smoke**

Smoking is quite hazardous for your skin. It causes wrinkles to form much earlier in your life. Smoking also narrows the blood vessels in the outermost layer of your skin, making your skin look a lot paler. It deprives your skin of all the nutrients needed to look healthier. So you must try to quit smoking. If you are a chain smoker and find it very hard to do that, you must try limiting it as much as your cancer. Apart from that, smoking is also known to be one of the causes of skin cancer. So you must try to limit your use. It won't happen all at once, but you can surely get there bit by bit. You can also ask your doctor to give you some useful tips to quit smoking.

- **Cut Back on Alcohol**

It would help if you cut back on your alcohol intake. Consuming excess alcohol is very bad for your skin. It increases your risk of developing different types of skin cancers. So it would help if you try to reduce your alcohol intake as much as possible. Again, it won't happen immediately, but you can try to cut back slowly and gradually. When you do that, you will see how your skin immediately feels rejuvenated and revived with time.

- **Stress**

Stress has the worst effect on your skin ever. It can cause acne breakouts and many other skin problems if left uncontrolled. So it would help if you tried to manage your stress levels at all times. Research has shown that stress can aggravate psoriasis and eczema too. There is an entire chapter in this book related to stress. Here, the question arises, what should one do to avoid stress? You can try different stress management techniques and see which works for you. If something is bothering you, then you must try to address the issue at the soonest. Try to consciously make an effort to block all thoughts that are stressing you out.

- **Get Ample Rest**

You must get rest. It shows up on your skin when you tire yourself beyond a certain point. Your skin looks saggy and extremely worn out. So try to focus on your sleep. Give your body the rest that it needs, and you will see all of it showing up on your skin very well. When you sleep, the blood flow to your skin improves, which allows you to have healthier and glowing skin. Astarita, a skin expert, talks about ample sleep for glowing skin. She says, "During sleep is when the body rests and regenerates through the elimination and replacement of dead cells, including skin and blood cells. More sleep also lowers the levels of the stress hormone cortisol, which causes free-radical damage to the skin and other systems in the body."

- **Exercise Regularly**

By now, you can see that exercising and staying active are directly related to keeping you healthy. The same is true for your skin, as well. When you exercise, the blood flow in your body increases, and your skin thus gets all the nutrients it needs. So, it would be best to try a healthy workout routine. When you do that, you will see how fresh your skin looks.

With all these skin care tips, you will surely have more youthful-looking skin! Try to make your skin a priority, and you will also see it showing up on your skin when you do that. However, if you have skin problems that have been persistent for a very long, then don't sit on them. This is your worst mistake and will only aggravate these skin problems. So try to make your skin a priority.

You must instantly visit a dermatologist to check your skin if you need to. Discuss your skin issues with them at length, and then follow through with what they say to ensure that your skin does well. Remember that your health is your responsibility. If you take it lightly, it will show up. To have youthful-looking skin, you must always start young. When you grow older, there isn't much you can do. So in your youthful days, try to be more responsible and prioritize your skin to avoid having saggy skin in the future.

As you age, skin problems may start becoming more common for you. You need to be the one to start taking care of your skin young, and you will see how it works out for you in the future!

Hair Loss and Aging

As you grow older, there are evident changes that you will see in your body. Just as you will see signs of aging in your skin, you will also see changes in your hair. For the most part, this can cause worry for many people, who will see how their physical appearance is affected by how their hair is changing. For those who are very conscious about their looks, hair loss and thinning can cause great distress to them.

Again, the idea here is to focus on how aging is a normal part of life, and there is no way to stop the process. However, the only thing that we can do is to understand how to deal well with it. Hair problems are also included in this. To better understand why you may experience hair changes, it would be useful to know more about your hair and what they are made up of.

Hair is made of protein strands. Your hair strand has a life of around two to seven years. Every year, your hair grows by about six inches. The factors that play a huge role in the overall health of your hair include diet, genetics, and age. As you age, the lifecycle of your hair becomes shorter and finer too. New finer hair replaces the older ones. Most people experience hair issues as they age. But you need to understand that this is a normal part of aging. As you age, many different changes happen in your body, including changes in your health and other nutritional changes. These then play a huge part in the way that your hair changes. As you age, some follicles might become weak, so they may not produce new hair. The hair fibers might also become thinner, and at times, they might never even regenerate.

You might even notice that your hair starts changing color at other times. It is quite common to see people have white hair as they age. Why is that so? The pigment cells in your hair stop producing as much as they once did, which is why you tend to lose your original hair color. Many people struggle with this issue, which is why you will see so many people use hair color. For women, menopause also brings many changes in their bodies, which is why they might see massive hair changes.

Different people see different changes in their hair. Some experience hair loss, others experience hair thinning, and some even experience their hair changing color. Some even experience all of this together. So if you are in the same boat, you don't need to worry since this is a normal part of aging. It affects everyone in different ways.

Symptoms

Here are a few symptoms that can tell you that you are suffering from hair problems and that you need to start doing something about it.

- **Gradual Thinning**

If you see your hair getting thinner from any part of the head, it should tell you that you are facing hair issues. Many people see this thinning happening right on the hairline. Some people even see it in the form of a receding hairline.

- **Bald Spots**

You might even start seeing bald spots on some parts of your head. These can be visible when they are on the front of the head. Sometimes, these can even be very itchy.

- **Hair Loosening**

Sometimes, you might even see that as you brush your hair, you see hair falling out all at once. This should show that your hair is getting looser from the roots, which is why they fall off easily.

So if you see any of these changes in your hair, you should begin taking steps to better deal with the whole process. You must take prompt steps as this is very important and may cause trouble if left unnoticed. While nothing you do guarantees you won't face hair issues, it will surely help you deal with the entire process much better.

Tips to Deal with Hair Loss

Dealing with hair loss can be quite stressful. This is especially true for those who experience hair loss to quite a great extent. However, here are a few tips that can be useful for all those suffering.

- **Focus on Your Diet**

The most important thing you should do is to focus on what you eat. What you take in your body has a profound impact on your hair. So to deal with it better, try to have a protein-rich diet. This will allow you to deal better with any nutritional deficiencies affecting your body. Try to avoid crash or fad diets as much as you can. This deprives your body of ample nutrition, which is, in fact, the leading cause of hair loss. People trying to shed extra kilos often complain that this affects their hair. So if you are trying to manage hair loss, try to focus on ensuring that your body gets ample nutrients and that you don't have to deprive your body of anything.

- **Wash and Condition Gently**

When washing your hair, try to use shampoos that don't have a lot of chemicals. Many people are recommended to use Sulfate-free shampoo. When you use shampoos with harsh chemicals, it can affect your hair in negative ways. So do your research and find mild shampoos that aren't very harsh for your scalp or overall hair health. Shampoos that are too harsh might rip your hair off all its moisture, which can also lead to hair loss.

After you wash your hair, make it a point to condition them. This allows your hair to retain moisture and remain soft. After you wash your hair, wrap them in a microfiber towel. This allows your hair to dry up quickly. How you wash and dry your hair weighs a lot on the overall well-being of your hair.

- **Avoid Washing Your Hair Every Day**

While it is recommended that you wash your hair enough to help you stay clean, experts recommend that you shouldn't wash your hair every day. While it does remove dirt and sweat from your hair, it also rids your hair of sebum, which is very important for hair growth. Sebum is a natural oil that makes it much easier for you to maintain your hair and for you to be able to have shiny hair. However, too much sebum also gives your hair a very greasy look. So you must always try to wash your hair once in two days. That allows for healthier hair without completely stripping it of its natural oil. This is highly advisable since it will allow your hair to become much better on the whole.

- **Avoid Blow Drying After Every Wash**

Some people blow-dry their hair after every wash. This can harm the hair and can also damage the roots. The damage that can do is massive. So, if you are dealing with hair loss, try not to over-expose your hair to eat. Instead, try to let your hair dry out naturally. When you do that, you will see changes in how your hair reacts. You can even towel dry your hair. This surely takes much more time but will help you deal with hair loss better.

- **Oil Your Hair Less Frequently**

While it is true that oiling your hair allows it to retain its moisture, try to keep that to a bare minimum. Contrary to popular belief, hot oil treatments weaken your roots and make your hair fragile, allowing them to break more frequently. When you oil your hair, try to be very gentle with them. Don't be too harsh with your hair. Rubbing the oil in your hair too much can lead to extra breakage, which might contribute to hair loss. So try to be as gentle as you can with your hair.

- **Brush and Comb Gently**

Sometimes, we tend to brush and comb harshly too. This is especially true if we have many tangles in our hair. Brushing and combing very hard can also lead to massive hair loss. So be as gentle as you can. Even if you have knots in your hair at certain places, try to get rid of them gently. In an attempt to save some time, most people tend to be very harsh when brushing their hair, which is the root cause of all problems. Never tug on your hair when you try to get rid of the knots.

- **Change Your Habits**

Many people have a habit of slowly tugging their hair or twisting it around. If you have any such habit, you should try to change your ways. While it doesn't seem like it is causing much damage, it is surely leading to many issues. In most cases, you might be doing it subconsciously, but it is also breaking your hair and causing other hair issues. So try to minimize that as much as you can.

- **Stop Styling Often**

Most people often use curling irons, flat irons, and hot combs. This is especially for socialites who often try to remain on top of their game and want their hair to look great at all times. You need to understand that styling your hair often overexposes them to heat, which can cause many issues later on. Try to minimize the use of these so your hair can grow healthy. When you style your hair very often, unnecessary tugging and pulling happen, which also affects hair health and leads to hair loss. So try to limit it as much as you can. You can surely style your hair on special occasions, but don't make it something you do every day.

- **Avoid Tying Your Hair Tightly**

Try to avoid making tight pigtails at the back of your head. Tying your hair tightly in a bun, pony, or pigtail pulls on it and triggers hair loss, known as traction alopecia. So try to limit this as much as possible. When you tie your hair, do so loosely, and don't pull on them too much. When you pull very tightly, it only leads to greater problems and triggers hair loss.

- **Protect Your Hair While You Sleep**

Sometimes, the material of your pillows also greatly contributes to hair loss. Your hair might get entangled in the cloth, leading to severe breakage. For this purpose, you must also protect your hair while sleeping. Silk or satin pillowcases can cause massive damage to your hair by breaking them. Apart from that, when you sleep with wet hair, that also causes massive damage to your hair. When your hair is wet, they are in a very vulnerable condition. That is when you must protect them as much as possible. So for that purpose, you should

- **Protect Your Hair From the Sun**

Overexposure to heat can also damage your hair. So try to protect your hair from the ultraviolet rays of the sun. In the same way that extra sunlight can damage your skin, it can also damage your hair. So when going out in the sun, try to protect your hair by wearing a hair. Prolonged exposure to sunlight will lead to your hair heating up. If that happens someday, you could even try putting on some aloe vera gel on your hair to repair the damage that has been done.

Get a Trim

Sometimes, you might also need to get a fresh haircut. For example, if you have long hair, then split ends can be quite a problem and make your hair feel much more brittle. Not just that, but you might also feel like your hair isn't looking as fresh as it was. Trimming can help, and it can weigh down fresh hair growth. You can get in touch with your stylist, who can guide you well about what you should be doing and how that can help.

- **Stop Smoking**

As mentioned several times in this book, smoking does more damage to your body than you can imagine. It causes inflammation in your body, which leads to hair loss. So try to limit your intake of tobacco. If possible, try to quit smoking soon since it can adversely affect your body and lead to massive hair loss.

- **Take Supplements**

Supplements can help reduce hair loss to a very great extent. However, to a great extent, vitamin deficiency can lead to hair loss. Vitamins and minerals that can help in this regard include selenium, vitamin B, zinc, vitamin D, and iron. The best products are the ones that contain recommended daily amounts of vitamins every day. However, if you choose to take supplements to help with hair loss, you must first get in touch with a doctor who can guide you better.

All of these tips can help you with hair loss. However, if you feel like the damage is massive, that you need to do something about it, and that no such tips are working for you, then you should consult a doctor so that they can help you with this issue. Sometimes, there are underlying issues that you might not really be aware of. These include skin issues and even other health conditions. Only when these conditions are diagnosed can they be cured in the best possible way. So for that reason, it is imperative that you first get in touch with a doctor.

You can then take supplements or certain medications based on what the doctor prescribes. That will surely help you deal with these issues much better.

Hair Masks for Healthy Hair

If you feel like your hair is losing its shine, or they just aren't as healthy as they were at a point in your life, then it is advisable to try these tips and home remedies. While there is no scientific evidence to prove these to be a hundred percent efficient, some swear by them since they have worked for them and helped them deal with these issues greatly.

Made of simple ingredients readily available in your kitchen, these hair masks are surely worth a try.

- **Eggs and Curd Mask**

Apply an oil that suits your hair. Most experts highly recommend coconut oil. Mix one egg and two tablespoons of curd till you get that thick consistency that you are looking for. Once you have that, take each strand at a time and apply it to your hair gently. Massage your hair till you cover all your hair. Once that is done, leave it on your hair for around twenty to thirty minutes. Rinse it off, after which you can shampoo your hair. This allows your hair to regain that lost shine. You will automatically feel your hair looking much healthier and shiny all at once.

- **Aloe Vera Mask**

Aloe vera is known to have proven benefits for your skin and your hair. Mix five tablespoons of aloe vera with your conditioner, and apply it to your scalp and hair strands. Once you have applied it throughout, comb your hair gently. Leave it on for at least twenty minutes before washing it off. This works if you have damaged hair. It gives your hair a nice feel and allows you to moisturize it deeply from within. It gives your hair that silky texture that you feel is lacking in your hair.

- **Avocado and Banana Hair Mask**

Avocado has a very high content of vitamin E, which surely helps your hair look much thicker. If you are suffering tom hair loss, this is great for your hair and can work wonders when it comes to giving it the lovely texture you are looking for. Mash one avocado and one banana together. Make sure the banana is fully ripe. That will allow for better consistency and for both ingredients to gel well together. This will surely make the application much better as well. Massage it into your hair gently. Keep it on for thirty minutes, and then wash it off. You will see a visible difference in your hair and notice how it makes it much healthier. If you use this mask twice a week, you will surely see a drastic difference in your hair.

- **Coconut Lemon Mask**

Coconut oil is as it is known to be great for your hair. Heat some coconut oil and add half a lemon juice to make this mask. Also, apply a little bit of money to your hair. Make sure that you also apply it to your scalp. When you do that, you will see how it helps you nourish your hair. This might feel itchy initially, but it will surely help you make your hair much smoother. Let it rest for at least half an hour, and then wash your hair with shampoo. You will see how much it helps you with your hair. It also makes the roots of the hair much stronger.

- **Coconut Cream and Cocoa Powder Mask**

This mask is known to work wonders for thin hair. You can use this mask if you have thin hair and want to see regenerated hair growth. It boosts hair growth and also promotes greater blood circulation in your hair. Add five ounces of coconut cream and half a cup of cocoa powder to make this mask. You can also add in some cinnamon powder if you like. After that, whisk all the ingredients together till thick paste forms. Once you have a thick consistency, apply it to your hair generously. Make sure to apply it to your scalp as well. Leave it on for thirty minutes, and then rinse it off. You will see how much it benefits you and how it helps your hair growth as well.

- **Apple Cider Vinegar Mask**

You can try this mask if you have a flaky and itchy scalp, due to which you see hair falling often. Its acidic nature helps cleanse your scalp, promoting better hair growth. You must have one part apple cider vinegar and ten parts water for this. Mix all of that and apply it to wet hair. Ideally, shampoo your hair first, and then after that, apply this to your wet hair as a conditioner. Let it rest in your hair for only five minutes, then wash it off. You will see how much it benefits you over time. Make sure to rinse it well once done. It allows the hair to see much better growth overall.

- **Sugar and Olive Oil**

This is also a great mask for your hair. It is a great exfoliator and lets you let go of any build-up in your hair. It also has great moisturizing benefits for your hair. Add two tablespoons of sugar and five tablespoons of olive oil. Mix it all up well, but while you do that, make sure that the sugar doesn't dissolve entirely. The idea is to have solid granules to allow for better scrubbing. Once you have mixed it, apply it well to your hair. Let it remain for around five to ten minutes, then rinse it. Immediately shampoo it, and you will see how it works magic in your hair.

- **Oats, Almond Oil, and Milk Mask**

If you feel like your hair is lifeless and want to add more volume to your hair, then this mask is great for you. It gives your hair a great energizing boost and makes it appear much better. To make this mask, mix half a cup of oats and add two tablespoons of almond oil. Next, add half a cup of milk as well. When you have added all of it in, mix the ingredients well. The mixture should be very smooth and well-blended. Once you apply it to your hair, leave it for around thirty minutes. After you are done with that, shampoo it well. Then after that, condition your hair as well. You will see how it works for you.

- **Onion Juice Hair Mask**

Onion is known to have proven benefits for your hair. Take two to three onions, chop them, and put them in a grinder. Once you have onion juice, apply it to your scalp and leave it there for around thirty minutes. Many people worry that this might lead to some smell in their hair, which can be problematic later on. However, this is not true. If you shampoo your hair well, this should not be a problem. So, make this mask and apply it to the roots of your hair. After thirty minutes or so, wash it off. It will leave your hair feeling deeply conditioned. If you do this religiously three to four times a week, you will see a vast difference in your hair growth over time.

Depending on your hair type and what suits you, you can apply these masks to your hair and see the difference. But remember that none of this is magic. It all depends on what suits your hair type.

So with these useful tips in mind, you will surely be able to see a difference in your hair. While at it, remember that hair fall should not hit your self-esteem. You need to realize that this is a lifecycle and that we all have to age. We will all grow old someday and must bear with what comes with that. Hair fall is a very normal part of aging. Most people go through it. We can only learn to master different ways of managing hair fall well.

Nail Health and Aging

In the same way, you see changes in your skin as you age; your nails also change over time. But this doesn't mean everyone sees the same changes in their nails. For example, some experience nail cracking, while others notice their nails becoming hard. Therefore, before you learn how to work towards healthier nails, you must understand why your nails change as you age.

When you grow older, there is cell turnover in your body. This affects your skin, as well as your nails. Experts suggest that as the cell turnover slows down, nails become thicker. Unfortunately, some people experience changes, so their nails start breaking due to this thickness. So how can you work towards healthier nails as you age?

The truth is that this is a normal part of aging. So the more effort you put into it, the better you can maintain your nails over time.

Tips for Healthier Nails

- **Keep Your Nails Clean**

The first and most important thing is always to keep your nails clean. If dirt accumulates, instantly clean your nails and remove any dirt piling up. This can really help you with your nails, allowing you to grow them healthier.

- **Keep Your Nails Dry**

Extra exposure to water makes your nails brittle. So whenever you are washing the dishes or doing your clothes, try to wear gloves. This will protect your nails, preventing breakage. Of course, keeping your hand protected from the water is not always possible. But you must try to make as much of an effort as possible.

- **Stay Hydrated**

In order to take care of your health, you must drink ample water. Experts recommend at least eight to ten glasses of water a day. So make a conscious effort to meet this requirement. This has a direct relation to your nail health as well. Hydration affects your whole body and your nails the most. When you have enough water, your nails retain moisture and don't break off that easily.

- **Eat Healthily**

Try to have a balanced diet. Incorporate food from all groups in your diet. This will keep you healthy overall and help you strengthen your nails. An entire chapter in this book talks about the importance of nutrition in your life. So it would help if you stay focused on that.

- **Trim Your Nails Regularly**

Trim your nails often. When you let your nails grow extra long, you increase your chances of breaking them. If you break your nails often, then they get weaker over time. So, trim them often, depending on how fast you grow out your nails. When you do that, you will see a huge difference in your nail health. Some people grow their nails very often, which can take time for some. So you need to be one to decide how often you should trim them off.

- **Don't Wear Very Tight Footwear**

When you wear extremely tight footwear, you end up damaging your nails. In addition, it can put extra pressure on your nails, causing them to break. So choose footwear that is comfortable for you. This is especially very important for your daily footwear. The more comfortable they are, the fewer you are breaking your nails.

- **Moisturize Your Nails**

After you wash your hand, try to rub moisturizer on your nails. This will help you keep your nails soft. This is especially very important if you have dehydrated nails. In addition, this prevents your nails from breaking. It would help if you make this a part of your nail care routine, and you will see how it helps you maintain your nails.

- **Don't Bite Your Nails**

If you have a habit of biting your nails, try to avoid it as much as possible. When you bite your nails, they don't grow out faster and become brittle over time. Sometimes, when you are nervous, you subconsciously start biting your nails. So try to work on this. First, make a conscious effort to stop yourself from biting your nails.

- **Never Ignore Nail Problems**

If you have any problems with your nails, never ignore them. If you just sit over your problems, they will only get worse with time. If you have an issue with your nails, visit a professional to help you. When you get your pedicures and manicures done, visit certified places to ensure you can trust them with your nails. This is extremely crucial and will allow you to provide healthy nails.

- **Use the Right Products**

If you use some nail products, use the right ones for your nails. These products should be certified and should be ones that suit you well. Don't rely on word of mouth to choose what you use for your nails. This can be very damaging and cause more damage to your nails than you think. When applying nail color, use nontoxic ones to avoid damaging your nails. When you use a nail color remover, try an acetone-free one.

- **Don't Use Gel or Acrylic Nails**

Some people love using gel or acrylic nails. At that time, they might seem very appealing to you. But the damage they do to your nails in the future is massive. So try to avoid using them as much as you can. Once in a while is no problem, but try not to make it a usual practice because it will only damage your nails further.

- **Never Pull Off Your Hang Nails**

Hangnails can be quite annoying. They don't just look distraught but can also cause a lot of pain. So if you ever see any hangnails, it is better to cut them off than pull them out. Pulling them out can even cause an infection, which is very harmful to you. So you must always be mindful of that.

- **Have Supplements**

Taking nail supplements can support nail growth and can also help make your nails much stronger over time. Biotin is an excellent supplement for your nails. It is water soluble and is known to have proven effects on your nails. Not just that, but it also helps the nervous system of the body to function well. Before you get a supplement for your nails, you need to ensure that it is safe for you, so get in touch with your health practitioner before you buy it.

- **Don't Use Your Nail to Do Things**

More often than not, we get lazy and use our nails for things we do. For example, you might use your nails to scratch a card or scrape some extra paint off. Unfortunately, that damages your nails and can cause breakage and chipping. So you must always be mindful of that because it can weaken your nail in the long run and cause immense pain.

- **Be Careful When Filing**

If you file your nails by moving in one direction, stop doing that entirely. When you do that, you ruin your nails and make them weaker. Instead, try to file them by moving them back and forth. Also, go very easy on the sides of your nails so they don't get weak with time.

- **Pay Close Attention to Your Shampoo**

Sometimes, chemicals in your shampoo can cause your nails to become extra dry, eventually weakening them and allowing them to break. So pay close attention to the shampoo that you are using. Try to use shampoos that don't strip off oil from your hair. You could even try to change your shampoo for a few weeks to see the difference.

- **Speak to your Doctor**

If you have tried multiple remedies and your nails still seem extra fragile and you notice them breaking often, you should get in touch with your doctor. He might prescribe some tests to see what is going on in your body, only after which he can prescribe a treatment that can strengthen your nails.

With these valuable tips, you can improve your nail health and make your nails much stronger. With age, like several other changes in your body, changes in your nails will also clearly be there. So don't fret over it too much. Instead, focus on your nail health and try to use these tips, and you will surely see a difference over time.

Memory Loss and Aging

We've all forgotten people's names, where we placed our house keys or someone's phone number. When we're younger, these things don't bother us as much. But as we age, we start to think about what these things might mean. We focus more on them, which makes us more worried. Memory loss usually comes as we age. Physiological changes might cause glitches in the brain, which means that recalling information might seem hard, and we may even see our cognitive abilities weaken. It is hard to say that this should not trouble you. Looking at yourself as unable to do things you could do when younger surely affects your mental health. But then, certain brain-related changes are inevitable. We can learn how to deal with them better and reduce the chances of these things happening to us.

Before you understand how to deal with memory issues, you must first understand that memory loss is not an inevitable result of aging. Your brain can produce new cells at any age. Many factors affect your ability to retain information and understand things in a better way. Some people confuse normal forgetfulness with dementia. You must understand that dementia is a medically diagnosed illness that is not the same as occasional forgetfulness. If you occasionally forget where you left your keys or the name of the person you met a few days back, you need to understand that this is normal. There is nothing to worry about. However, you can learn how to deal with this better way. Dementia can be disabling, but age-related memory loss sure isn't. While memory lapses might affect your daily performance, you won't see that drastic effect if you notice that memory loss has become pervasive and only worsens with time; you need to visit a doctor to get checked.

Before learning more about helpful tips that can help you deal with dementia better, it would be useful to understand what all age-related memory loss entails. If you are facing all the following, then chances are that you are suffering from age-related memory loss:

- Occasionally forgetting things like where you kept the keys
- Being able to recall incidents where you forgot things
- Usually, forget directions but can recall them after thinking about it
- Find it difficult to recall the right words sometimes
- Judgment and decision-making ability aren't harmed to a very great extent

You don't need to worry if you suffer from some or all of the above. Age-related memory loss is quite normal. There are also many ways that you can help improve your memory.

Tips to Improve Your Memory

Here are a few useful tips that can help you improve your memory:

- **Remain Physically Active**

This book has an entire chapter on the importance of physical activity only because it is essential for healthy aging. When you exercise, the blood flow to your whole body increases, including your brain. This can play a part in helping you keep your memory sharp. You can indulge in any form of physical activity you like if you keep active. Try to spare some time in a day and indulge in anything that makes your pulse go up.

- **Remain Mentally Active**

Staying mentally active is just as important as being physically active. What does being mentally active mean? It means that you don't remain idle. You always need to have something to do. If you don't have much on your plate, then find something to do that stimulates brain activity. When your brain keeps working and you remain occupied doing something important, you will see how it helps you remain sharp. A few things you could do is solve puzzles or play any other games in which cognitive activity is involved.

This will only help you get sharper. The more you use your brain, the stronger it tends to get.

- **Learn Something New**

Learning something new takes quite some energy. You need to continuously keep your brain challenged to function at optimum capacity. So try to learn new things. Try it even if you must step out of your comfort zone to do that. You could try learning how to play a new instrument. You could even learn something like making pottery or a new language. It will surely not be easy to do, but if it challenges you mentally, it is helping you make your brain more robust, which is what you need.

- **Meditate**

Meditation allows you to relax. It allows you to let go of whatever is bothering you. As a result, when you meditate, you will naturally feel much calmer, which means that you can sharpen your mind and automatically see your memory improving too.

- **Elaborate and Rehearse**

Every time you try to retain something, you could try to repeat it and consciously try to remember it too. This can help you retain information. Elaborative rehearsal is also one of the most effective coding techniques that allow things to go into your long-term memory. That way, you can remember things for longer. When you do this, you will see that remembering things will automatically seem much easier.

- **Visualize**

Whenever you want to remember something, try to visualize it. Pay attention to any photographs or anything you can remember related to that. When you picture things, your chances of remembering those become much higher.

- **Organize Yourself**

When you're organized, things will automatically start seeming very orderly. It helps you sort things out properly as well. Jot down all the important things that you have to do. Have a to-do list too, and you will see how it becomes easier to remember things. Also, limit all distractions. All this will surely help you stay calmer, allowing you to remember things fully.

- **Focus**

Try to give it your utmost focus whenever you want to remember something. This will help you retain it. You could even connect it to a song or a smell. These two bring back memories. So when you consciously try to remember, things will automatically start falling into place for you.

- **Pay Extra Attention to Difficult Things**

You are more likely to forget things when you don't understand them well. So if there is something you can't understand well or are struggling to make sense of, try to pay extra attention to that. Spend the extra time trying to focus on what is being said, and you will see how much it helps you focus, allowing you to remember later.

- **Socialize**

Social Interaction is extremely important for older adults, as mentioned earlier. It allows you to feel that sense of connection and also allows you to remain fresh and active. Speaking to other people wards off feelings of loneliness and glumness and makes you feel worthy. So try to connect with those around you. It can be friends, distant family, neighbors, etc. But be in the company of those who genuinely make you happy and those whom you can enjoy with. When you do that, you will see that it will positively affect your mind, allowing you to connect better with your inner self and your being. When you feel fresher, you remain mentally active too, which is very important and thus allows you to remember things better.

- **Sleep Well**

The importance of sound sleep every night cannot be stressed enough. There is an entire chapter in this book that covers the importance of sleeping well. When you sleep well, you allow your mind to shut off completely. You allow your body to get the rest it needs to function fully. That eventually helps you relax and allows your brain to function well. It allows you to remember things well too. When you're sleep-deprived, you will find yourself struggling to focus too. Make your sleep schedule, depending on what works for you, and then stick to it. You will see how much it affects your life and allows you to function in the best possible way.

- **Limit Alcohol Intake**

Alcohol does nothing good for your body. It harms your health in many ways, so you must limit its intake. Studies have shown that it harms the brain and its functioning as well. If you drink a certain amount daily, try to minimize your intake one day at a time. Take it slow and steady, but consume as little as possible. You will be amazed to see the effect it has on memory function.

- **Chunk Information**

There are several tactics for remembering things, and chunking is also one of them. You can break things down into pieces or chunks, making it much easier for your brain to remember. Clubbing things together simplifies them, and your brain then doesn't have to work as hard remembering. For example, if there is a number 094827639, you could probably make chunks like 094-827-639. Breaking it down this way will help you remember it much better.

- **Rely Less on Technology**

While technology has allowed us to simplify our lives in many ways, it has also made us increasingly dependent. For example, ever since Google Maps came up, we don't make as much effort as we should to remember things. Technology has made us lazy. It has allowed us to understand that there are ways of going about things without using our brains. So this is something that we must be wary of. Try to remember things without depending too much on technology. You will see how much simpler your life becomes. If someone tries to explain something to you, try remembering it instead of being lazy and turning to Google as the need arises. If we want to make the best use of technology, we must use it sensibly. Otherwise, it allows our brain to function at a very low capacity, which is detrimental to us.

- **Focus on Nutrition**

An entire chapter is dedicated to nutrition and its effect on your life. Nutrition is also very important for your memory. Foods that can help you make your brain stronger include whole grains, legumes, nuts, fish, olive oil, and fish. Try to avoid sugar and processed foods as much as you can. You will see how it helps you a lot in your life. Not only will you feel much healthier, but you will also see an instant effect on your memory retention.

- **Increase Water Intake**

Ample water intake is very important for you! You must try to have at least ten glasses of water each day. Memory loss also has a lot to do with dehydration. So, the more water you have, the better fueled your brain is to function at its utmost capacity. So, even if you aren't thirsty, try to drink more water. You will see how much it helps you with time.

- **Avoid Certain Medications**

Some medicines might give you instant relief but aren't good for you in the long run. These tend to affect how your brain functions, making it difficult to retain things. Examples include anti-depressants, sleeping pills, and hypertension drugs. Try to avoid these as much as you can unless necessary. This is very important and allows you to become more self-reliant. Instead, focus more on natural things as much as you can.

Now that you know how to improve your memory, you should start the process immediately.

The next question that might come to your mind is, how do you know when to see the doctor?

When to See a Doctor?

As mentioned, memory loss usually comes with aging. But when should you be greatly concerned? If the memory lapses become more frequent and start affecting your daily activities that is when it should be alarming. You should get an appointment with the doctor immediately and check yourself to see the problem. Even if you don't have all the symptoms of dementia, it is always better to take preventive measures early on. This only stops the problem from becoming a bigger one. So the sooner you take action, the better it is.

Your doctor can check you to see all personal risk factors. They can also evaluate your symptoms to see where you lack and eliminate all causes of memory loss. They will also ensure that you get the proper care you need. Early diagnosis can help prevent further damage that may be irreversible if you find out much later in life. When examining you, the doctor might ask many questions about how often you forget things or what things you find hard to remember. This will help them better diagnose your condition. Once they correctly diagnose the issue, they can provide you with the necessary care and prescribe certain medications.

Sex and Aging

Sexual health is important for all ages. However, like most other things, you also experience changes in your sex life as you age. As you age, your body changes, and so do your body requirements. This means that there are many different things that you may experience as you age. In addition, aging brings transitions that create opportunities for older adults to redefine what sexuality means to them.

If you are experiencing changes in your sex drive as you age, then that is nothing you should be worried about. It is completely normal. The good part about it is that you can work on it; with time, you will surely see a positive change in your sex life. However, before we move on to the different ways to help improve our sex lives, we must first understand what these expected changes are.

Expected Changes

Sexuality has a direct connection to one's emotional and physical state. Your physical state affects your ability to do something, whereas your mental state affects what you might want to do. Many older people complain that they found greater satisfaction when they had sex as younger people and feel that their sexual drive has significantly decreased. Some even complain that they get tired much sooner. They also talk about how they had lesser worries when they were younger and didn't have to worry about getting pregnant, which is why they also enjoyed sex much more. Others complain that they find it hard to form that connection with their spouse that leads to greater intimacy and eventually sex.

Here the most important thing to understand is that your body changes as you age, which massively affects your ability to enjoy sex. This includes changes in body weight, skin, and muscle. Some older people even complain that they aren't as comfortable in their bodies as they once were. They sometimes also feel that their partner might not find them attractive anymore due to how their body has changed.

Most older adults also experience great changes in their sex organs. For men, it is common to experience erectile dysfunction as they age. This means that they might not be able to keep an erection for long, or the erection might not be as firm as it once used to be. While this is not a very big problem if it happens seldom. However, you might need to consult a doctor if you see it happening every often.

For females, it is common to experience thinning of the vaginal walls. Sometimes, you may even notice that the vaginal walls become stiffer and that there is much lesser vaginal lubrication. For this reason, penetration can be less desirable or even painful in some situations. Another huge factor that affects sexuality in females is menopause. The menopausal transition can last for some years and is only considered to stop when a woman hasn't had a period in one year. In this entire phase, she might see many changes in herself. These include hot flashes and trouble falling asleep. There are different therapies that doctors use to help deal with menopause in a better way. Due to these menopausal symptoms, women tend to experience a lowered sex drive.

Other factors affecting sex in older adults include chronic issues like diabetes, body aches, dementia, depression, alcohol addiction, obesity, etc. However, the good news is that you can work on this and can improve your sexual health as you age. No matter what your age, to keep the spark in your relationship alive, you must work on your sex life. A lot of the satisfaction in your marriage comes from your physical relationship with your spouse. So you must work on it.

Benefits of Sex as You Age

Sex has proven benefits when it comes to your personal life. It can allow you to improve your mental and physical health manifold. When you have sex, your brain releases endorphins, instantly making you feel better and reducing your anxiety. Research has also shown that sex increases your lifespan. When you age, your spouse is the one you must lean on, no matter how much everyone claims to love or care for you, your spouse will be the only one, who will be with you till the very end. Your kids are busy in their own lives, so this is the time that you can solidify your relationship with your spouse, and sex helps you do just that.

Maintaining a Satisfying Sex Life

Contrary to popular belief, you can easily maintain a satisfying sex life as you age. Here are a few ways to work on your sex life as you age.

- **Communicate**

The most important thing is to communicate with your partner. If you feel certain changes are happening with your body, try to speak about it openly with your partner. In a marriage, the last thing you should do is keep things from each other. So always speak about how you feel, what is making you uncomfortable, and what helps you increase intimacy. If there is something that stimulates you better, let your partner know so that you can both work on improving the intimacy that you have with each other. Understand that it is completely normal to feel vulnerable. Only once you talk to each other can you build the relationship you want. Communication is the key to leading a healthy sex life.

- **Visit a Healthcare Provider**

If something is wrong with your body, or if you feel like physical changes are making you uncomfortable, instantly visit a healthcare provider and discuss your issues. They can help you manage long-term chronic conditions, which is very important to help you keep the spark alive in your sex life. If you're concerned about your testosterone levels, it is also wise to ask a healthcare provider for guidance who can take you through the entire process.

- **Counseling**

You can also speak to a counselor about what is bothering you. Sexual health counselors can help you resolve all of your issues. First, you need to tell them what is bothering you- if certain mental or emotional factors are causing a hindrance in your sex life, then you and your partner must both get counscling to help you overcome those issues. You can even discuss other aging concerns with them, and they will surely help you find your way through all of those issues.

- **Exercise Regularly**

Regular exercise helps you with your sex life, too, just as it does with all of your other health conditions. It helps you strengthen your muscles, which means you won't have to worry about hurting your back or pulling a muscle. Sex also has a direct relation to your mood. Exercising instantly helps lift your mood, making you much more comfortable. Furthermore, it helps you become the fittest version of yourself. That eventually helps boost your confidence and, ultimately, your sex life. Men who are relatively more active are less likely to have erectile dysfunction issues. So you can start off with any exercise that works for you.

- **Build Up**

Don't just jump straight to intercourse. If you do so, it will only cause pain to you and your spouse. Before doing anything make sure you are considering your spouse's consent because it is the most important thing to notice before getting intimate with your spouse. There are others options you have that can help you enjoy closeness and pleasure.

- **Get Comfortable**

One of the most important things is for you to get comfortable. It will undoubtedly lead to a compromised experience if you aren't comfortable.

- **Wait for Recovery**

Give your body time to recover if you have gone through some serious illness or injury. Jumping straight into sex might make things very difficult for you. So start very slowly at first. Speak to your partner about how you're feeling and how your injury affects you.

- **Set Aside Time for Sex**

Make a conscious effort to set aside some time for sex. When you put aside some time for sex, it allows you to nurture your relationship and foster intimacy.

With these few tips, you can improve your sex life manifold. This allows you to work on your relationship and keep that spark alive! The idea is to find out what works for you and then stick to that. Every person has individual bodily needs, so you must never compare yourself to another. Always focus on yourself and how you feel. Tailor your needs based on your own requirements, and then work towards getting just that. These tips will surely allow you to make the most of your sex life, as you age.

Debunking Aging Myths

We've all heard about aging myths- notions that we believe to be true, but any solid evidence doesn't back them up. They are rampant in our culture and have distorted our understanding of aging. Unfortunately, these popular aging misconceptions have distorted our understanding of the concept of aging.

In this chapter, the idea is to debunk these aging myths to better understand the concept of aging and how it works.

1. Depression comes with aging.

While it is very common for older adults to face depression, it is not a normal part of aging. Growing older means that you tend to see a lot of changes in your life that might not be positive. For example, you might see people your age dying, you might start finding yourself useless after retirement, or you might even face multiple health issues. These factors can have a major impact on how you feel and can make you depressed. But this doesn't mean that everyone faces depression as they age. However, those who do face depression need to get treatment for it at the soonest, especially if it starts impairing normal functioning. In addition, the stigma associated with depression needs to be discussed more, and people need to realize why it is important to speak about what bothers them openly or seek professional help as needed.

2. Older people should limit physical exercise.

In many cultures across the world, people still believe that you should limit physical exercise as much as possible as you age. They believe that your bones become frail as you age, which means that you should limit physical activity so that you don't exert too much pressure on your bones. Some also believe that you should avoid exercising to prevent the risk of injury or to keep yourself from falling. This is the farthest thing from being true. Exercising only makes you stronger and also much more active. It helps you fight off so many diseases and also instantly lifts your mood. In this book, time and again, the importance of exercise has been stressed. So you already know how beneficial exercise is for your overall health and how it can help you boost your immune system too.

3.   Older people need less sleep.

With old age, you might have a hard time trying to fall asleep. Due to this, many people believe that your sleep needs decline as you age. The truth is that you should sleep as much as your body requires. For some, this can be seven hours, but for some, this can even be ten hours. So depending on your physical condition and your bodily needs, you will require sleep. Adequate sleep helps you function well and also helps you reduce your risk of falling. So depending on several factors affecting your health, you need to figure out how many hours of sleep works for you.

4.   Older people can't learn new things.

Many people believe that older adults cannot learn new things due to declining cognitive ability and memory impairment. Learning is a lifelong process that only ends as you die. When you try to learn new things, it can help you improve your cognitive abilities manifold and also helps you stay busy doing things you like. So you must always try to keep learning new things as you age. This can be anything at all that helps you remain engaged and allows you to wipe your boredom away. Learning new things helps makes your memory sharper and allows you to become a much better version of yourself. When you remain engaged in doing something productive, it is only a step forward that helps you improve your brain functioning.

5.   Older people should give up driving.

Many believe that they should give up driving as they age. While it is true that natural physical changes in your body may affect you in different ways, like that having a slower response rate or diminished vision, that doesn't mean that you need to put a stop to driving. Aging is normal, so you don't have to give up on all you used to do as you age. It only means that you should keep a check and only drive if you are comfortable with it. You can speak with your doctor, who can guide you better in this regard. But remember, safety always comes first- not just your own but also of those on the road. So always make sure that you take the necessary precaution when driving, and practice patience as you do too.

6. Older people should quit smoking.

Many believe that quitting smoking as you age is impossible. They believe that addiction becomes very strong as you age, so quitting becomes near impossible. The truth is that you can do anything that you set your mind to. You are never 'too old' to do anything. When you quit smoking, you will notice your life's much better. You will see so many positive changes in your life when you quit smoking. It enhances feelings of overall well-being too. You will see the benefits of quitting smoking almost immediately. It improves the quality of your life manifold too. So if you think you are too old to quit smoking, change that mindset and work on yourself to improve your life.

7. Older people are unhappy.

Many people believe that unhappiness is bound to come with old age. While seniors do sometimes feel discontent, it is not something that affects everyone. Some people don't deal well with major life changes. They feel like their life is falling apart, and they don't have the things that they once used to. This makes them unhappy. But others deal with everything very well and simply enjoy their free time the way they want.

8. Older people have limited family interaction.

Again, this is a very popular misconception. Sometimes, people choose to cut themselves off from others. But this is not true for everyone. Sometimes, people have more family interaction when they are older because they have more spare time and can spend their time the way they like.

9. Older people are cranky.

The "grumpy old people" stereotype has been there for years and is extremely damaging. While it is true that some older people don't know how to deal with their emotions well and lose their calm when something doesn't go their way, it is also true that this doesn't happen to everyone. Those who are cranky suffer from chronic health conditions and cognitive decline in most cases. On the other hand, the comparatively healthier ones are seen to be more trusting and good-natured. They enjoy their own company and live the lives of others around them.

10. Older adults have many regrets.

Not everyone regrets things they have done in their lives. Instead, many take their shortcomings simply as learning experiences that allow them to grow. These learning experiences allow them to boost their overall outlook on life.

11. Only older females need to be worried about osteoporosis.

Osteoporosis is more common in women, but men also have a chance of suffering from it. For this reason, both men and women need to start caring for their bones from a very young age. The same factors that put men at risk of suffering from this problem also put women at risk. This means that both have to be equally concerned.

12. If a family member has Alzheimer's disease, it will be passed on.

This is not true at all. While one of the factors affecting the risk of developing Alzheimer's is genetics, it is not the only factor. However, you need to start working on this to ensure that you aren't at a very high risk of developing this problem. Factors that affect this include exercise, diet, and lifestyle as well. So you need to try to limit your chances of having this disease by focusing on the above factors.

13. Older people should expect falls as they age.

Older adults are more prone to falling. This is true, but that doesn't mean that you should expect to fall as you age. If you are cautious and take good care of yourself, you will not fall. You just need to be extra careful about this. Falling at an older age puts you at risk of developing many problems. So you need to be one to take extra care of this. Strength and balance exercises allow you to minimize your risk of injury from falling. You need to take extra care by removing anything you might have on the floor that increases your risk of falling.

14. Older people need others to make healthcare decisions for them.

In most cases, the children make healthcare decisions for their children. This is not important at all. If you wish to make your own healthcare decisions and have complete thinking capacity and are of sound mind, then you should make your own healthcare decisions. However, if you think you need extra help or advice from your loved ones, then there is no harm in seeking help from them. They will surely help you with what you need, and you will see yourself doing much better.

15. Older adults don't contribute much to household chores.

Many people believe that older adults idle their time away and barely contribute to household chores. This is also the farthest thing from being true. Older people have much more spare time on hand, which means that they can contribute more to household chores. It depends entirely on how they wish to proceed with things and whether or not they wish to help.

16. Older adults are ignorant.

Many people also feel that older people are much more ignorant and that they don't have a lot of knowledge about world affairs. Ignorance has nothing to do with your age. If you remain up-to-date with all that is happening, you can very well do that. Some seniors are very focused on finding out about things and engaging in debates focused on current affairs and world events.

17. Old age means no sex.

Your sex life can only be as interesting as you make it. So old age does not mean the end of sex. You can continue to enjoy sex even when older. In this book, an entire chapter talks about your sex life as you age and what you can do to make your sex life more enjoyable. Of course, your physical relations with your spouse are critical in helping you build that relationship in the best way possible. So you can also make your sex life more interesting as you age. It depends entirely on how you view things in your life.

18. You become dependent on others as you age.

Many believe that old age brings dependency- both financial and physical. This is true for some but not for all. You will only be as dependent as you make yourself. Many people save up their whole lives just so that they can support themselves as they age. However, some of them also work very hard on their physical selves to get what they want in life. So, it isn't a rule of thumb that old age brings with it a dependency. You are only as dependent as you make yourself. So, it is entirely up to you and depends on your outlook on life.

19. Old people don't need to get their vision checked often.

Weaker vision is one of the major factors that lead to many other issues in your life. Unfortunately, it also increases your chances of falling. So you need to be extremely careful about this. It is best that you get your vision checked every few months. This will help you focus on your health and will help you work your way through things.

20. Old age brings problems.

While it is true that you might experience a lot of issues with your physical health as you age, this is not true for everyone. Old age is not a problem at all. It depends entirely on how you work on your health. Some people are very healthy even when they age. So you need to be one to invest in your health. Make your health a priority; you will see how it bears fruit.

So these were a few common misconceptions that people have about old age. With these myths debunked, you can work better on yourself and not take old age as a problem.

The Virtue of Forgiveness

Stress and anxiety can cause more distress in your life than you can ever imagine. Older people have had several experiences with people throughout their lives, and not all of them have been positive. Some people have hurt them, which has caused them great distress. Due to this reason, they also hold grudges in their heart and find it very hard to forgive some people.

Forgiveness is a virtue. No matter how much someone has hurt you, you must always find it in your heart to forgive them. Of course, it is going to be hard. It is going to require much more heart than you could ever imagine. But holding grudges against people only makes you a bad person. It also causes great stress, leading to overall health issues. On forgiveness, Joyce Meyer says, "Forgiveness is not a feeling - it's a decision we make because we want to do what's right before God. It's a quality decision that won't be easy, and it may take time to get through the process, depending on the severity of the offense." I love this quote because it talks about how forgiveness is a decision we make that surely isn't easy. Yet, we must find it in ourselves to forgive others, not for them but for us. Just so that we can make our own lives a lot better. Will Smith also talks about forgiveness. He says, "Throughout life, people will make you mad, disrespect you, and treat you badly. Let God deal with their actions because hate in your heart will consume you too."

So learn to let go. It will help you make your own life so much better, allowing you to deal with everything that comes your way.

Tips to Forgive Others

Here are a few useful tips that will help you forgive others and will allow you to help you make your own life much better eventually.

- **Understand the Benefits**

To be able to forgive others and understand the countless benefits that it has. When you forgive others, you are essentially simplifying your own life, which is crucial to help make your own life better. You do not forgive them because they deserve it, but rather forgive them because you want to be able to feel better yourself. Holding grudges is not doing you any good either. It is only making you feel much worse and is making you very stressed too. So find it in yourself to understand that this is for your own good and will help you make your own life so much better. So do it for your own self, because your life matters.

- **Talk Through Your Feelings**

Sometimes, we find it very hard to understand ourselves and why we feel a certain way. So talk through your feelings and process all that you are going through. Understand why you are feeling a certain way. Understand how it is affecting you. Then, embrace those feelings and accept them. We often deny our feelings, which doesn't allow us to move on and understand things in the best way possible.

- **Look at the Bright Side**

Understand that when you forgive others, you will only be allowing yourself to purify your heart of your negative feelings. It will allow you to have a fresher perspective on life, eventually being able to make your life so much better. So try to understand why it is beneficial and how it will help you. Let's look at it this way: if someone in your family said something mean to you and hurt you. Try to understand how forgiving them will help you through so many things. It will help you improve your own life. It might also help you improve family relations. So try to look at the brighter side of things. When you only focus on the negative, it also makes you a very negative person. So focus on the good, and you will see how much simpler your own life becomes. Martin Luther King explained why forgiveness was important. He said, "We must develop and maintain the capacity to forgive. He who is devoid of the power to forgive is devoid of the power to love."

- **Try to Move On**

Often, we find ourselves stuck in a cycle where forgiving starts to seem impossible. We remain adamant about our stance and find it hard to move on from a certain position we had. This is very bad for your mental health. Try to move past things, and let things of the past remain in the past. Focusing too much on what happened once upon a time in the past only worsens your suffering. So you must try to move past that. When you do that, you will be able to see the good in things and will be able to understand things much better. Make a conscious effort to try and move past things because holding grudges will only make you more negative.

- **Try to Look at Their Good Side**

Try to focus on the good things that others have done for you. When you focus on that, you will be able to see the humanity in a much more positive light, which will eventually help you move on.

Planning for End of Life

The average lifespan in the world is 72.74 years. So it is only inevitable to think about our end as we age. The biggest truth is that we are all going to die one day. Yet, very few people give a thought to end-of-life planning. End-of-life planning isn't only for those who have huge financial assets in their name. It is for everyone so that your loved ones won't have to face the burden of managing your affairs once you're no more. It can be quite stressful to deal with all of what comes after you're gone, so you might as well make it easy for your loved ones. Not just that, but end-of-life planning also allows you to make sure that things are done your way when you are not there.

From the distribution of your financial assets to healthcare decisions, insurance policies, and online accounts, end-of-life planning encompasses it all. Bereaved family members can find it quite challenging to manage certain affairs alongside also dealing with such an immense loss. So it is only befitting for us to make the process a lot more manageable for them. Families who have struggled with the task of managing a deceased person's affairs know how challenging it can be.

For most people, end-of-life planning begins when they fall sick at an old age, once they cross a certain age, or once they see signs that tell them that they are about to die. But this is surely not the right approach. None of us knows how long we are going to live or what turn of events can come our way. So for that, we must focus on end-of-life planning well beforehand. We never know when our life can take an unexpected turn, so being ready before time is surely the best thing to do.

Points to Consider When Planning for End of Life

So, when you are planning for the times that you'll be no more, it is important to focus on some very important factors. In your lifetime, you must organize all of your affairs. The more sorted things are, the better they can be managed without you. Otherwise, your loved ones might have a very tough time dealing with all that comes. It is always best to have things in writing so that after you are gone, your loved ones don't have a hard time sorting things out. You first need to gather all the important documents like your birth certificate, social security number, employment records, medical papers, property papers, and any other documents you think are important and put them in a safe place. It is always ideal to choose a single location for all these important documents and let your family members know where they are.

Now I will explain what exactly you need to be mindful of, considering each factor separately.

- **Make a Will**

Most people make their will when they are old. Research has shown that 70% of Americans don't even have a will. This is quite shocking. It is very important to have a will so that your loved ones know what you want after you are not there anymore. While this is one of the most important things, there is, not many people know how to make a will. A common misconception is that making a will is expensive or time-consuming. This is not true at all. Having a will in place ensures no family conflicts once you're gone. Not just that, but it also allows others not to be confused about what they should be doing once you are not there.

To make a will, you must be anywhere above 18. You must also be of sound mind and have at least two witnesses who can confirm that you were under no stress at the time you made the will and that everything written in the will is solely your discretion. So now, how do you make a will?

- **Decide How You Will Make It**

A lot of people decide to take the legal route when making a will. They take a lawyer's help who gets them through the whole process with a lot of ease. However, many decide to make their wills themselves using different online platforms. So you need to first decide what route you will take. If you plan to make it yourself, the following steps can help you get through it easily.

- **Include Important Points**

While making your will, you must include important points that make your will valid. For example, you must make it very clear that this is your last will and that you are doing this with your discretion. This helps put things in place. It will make it very clear that you are doing all of this your own self.

- **Decide What Property to Include**

After people die, the one thing that causes more problems is the financial assets under their name and who they go to after the person dies. So you need to first decide which assets you will include in your will. If you have a lot of property in your name, you must list all of it down first. This includes your physical property as well as your financial assets. For example, your house, your car, your bank account, etc. You must make everything clear so no one can take advantage of anything after you.

- **Decide Who Gets What**

This is the part you need to pay attention to, especially if you have a lot of assets in your name. More often than not, this is what leads to most major family disputes. People aren't able to decide who gets what after the person dies, so you need to state it out very carefully in your will. First of all, write down which of your properties goes to whom. After you have made your first choice, also make sure to add alternate beneficiaries in case something goes wrong and your first choices aren't there to take all you had.

When you write down all of this, you need to make sure to write their names in full, alongside digits that can help identify them. Going into such detail might seem insignificant or more like a waste of time at this stage, but you don't know how important this is and how it can save your loved ones from so much confusion and quarrels later on. You must also have a residual beneficiary, who will receive all of the assets you didn't claim or give to anyone.

- **Choose an Executor**

Next, you need to choose someone who will make sure that what you write in your will is carried out. This person doesn't have to be someone like a lawyer. It can be anyone from your household who you trust. That person can later hire someone to get this done if they deem fit. You also need to ensure that the person you choose knows that you chose them for this. This is important so they can instantly take charge of things once you aren't there.

- **Choose a Guardian for Your Child**

You also need to choose a guardian for your children, especially if they are young. Who doesn't want their children to be raised in the right way? So you must choose an adult who you think is responsible enough to bring your children up well.

- **Find Witnesses**

You need to find two witnesses who know exactly what you are doing. These witnesses have to be people you trust and people who you know aren't manipulative so that the process can be carried out very well.

- **Print and Sign Your Will**

Once you have written all the necessary information, you must print and sign your will in front of your family and your witness. This will allow you to tell everyone that you have done the needful.

- **Keep It in a Safe Place**

Once you are done with the abovementioned points, make sure to keep your will in a safe place. Make sure your family members know where you are keeping it so they can access it easily in your absence.

Consequently, you can make it all very easy when you aren't there. This way, you can ensure that everything is done according to what you want.

For those with very complicated family dynamics or business owners, it is recommended that you get it all done through a lawyer. A lawyer knows how to deal with these things correctly and will make you much more at ease.

Have Difficult Conversations

It is very hard to imagine life without loved ones. But the truth is that we all have to go one day. You would much rather have things sorted out than just leave haywire when you aren't there. So you must have end-of-life conversations with your loved ones. You need to ensure that each of your family members is there when you have this conversation. Of course, it is going to be difficult, and there will be very difficult moments, but there is no way you can go without it either.

There is no particular rule about end-of-life conversations. They can sure be hard, so you must follow your instincts when doing so. Speak with those people who matter to you and the ones you feel most connected to. Make sure that you tell your loved ones that you want to speak to them out of choice and that this is very important to you.

There is nothing wrong with having end-of-live conversations. In fact, when you gather with people you value the most, you also get to know about their feelings. A study conducted about end-of-life discussions found that while 90% of people felt that it was very important to have these end-of-life conversations with people, very few actually had them. Only 27% of these people actually talked to their loved ones about the times they won't be there (Correll, 2021).

Many people try to run away from this ultimate truth. However, it is always sensible about every topic you have to go through in your life. When you have these discussions with your loved ones, try to make them understand that when you aren't in this world, they will have to be the ones who will take charge of everything. Try to make them know that it will not be easy, but they have to find it in them to muster up all the courage that they have in them and sort things out. When having this end-of-life discussion with your loved ones, make sure to discuss these important points:

Tell Them How Much You Love Them

Life is very short-lived, and more often than not, we never succeed in telling our loved ones how much we love them. You need to make sure that you tell your loved ones what they mean to you. When you do so, make sure that you do it on a very positive note, instead of having everyone lamenting. Tell them that this will happen and that there is no way they can try to control it. Tell them that while you may not be there with them some time down the road, your love will live on. Also, remember to cherish your time with your loved ones because you never know who will stay longer later on.

Forgive Them

If any of your family members has hurt you, forgive them for it. Tell them that while they may have hurt you, you have decided to move on and have no hard feelings against them. When you do that, you will see how nice it makes you feel and how it makes you feel so much better about your family relationships.

Sometimes, we end our relationship and water the selfishness rising within. However, when we forgive others and give them fair chances, they value us and understand their mistakes.

Once you start forgiving others, it will allow you to understand your family dynamics much better. When you have no hard feelings, you immediately feel less stressed and thus feel happiness and peace in your overall surroundings.

Advise Them

Try to give useful pieces of advice to your family members. Since this is a very serious discussion you are having with them, it will stick with them, and your advice will surely go a long way. Try to tell them about all that you have learned in this time and why it is so important. Share your wisdom with them. It is sure to go a very long way and will allow them to understand things much better. While advising the youngsters, make sure you are not imposing anything on them; if you do that, they will create distance from you and thus won't understand the lesson behind your advice.

Share Meaningful Moments with Them

When you talk to your loved ones about the end of life, also discuss the meaningful moments in your life, talking to them about what memories you cherish the most. Also, tell them why. When you do that, you will see how they will have so many positive things to remember when you aren't there. These are the memories that they will cherish and are ones that they will hold very dear to them as well.

Recognize and Resolve Conflicts

Make sure you recognize and resolve the conflicts in your family. If there are any hard feelings that your loved ones have with each other or any conflicts they are a part of, try to resolve them by acting as a mediator. That will surely cause a lot of emotional pain and distress, but that will allow you to play a very positive role in things. Try to focus on telling them how and why resolving conflicts is important and why this is something that they should be mindful of.

We often avoid talking about certain things and hurt each other without any specific cause. Make sure you are the one who takes over the lead and handle everything perfectly. When resolving conflicts, also tell them why you think it is important for them to understand what you want after you die. Tell them why the last thing you want from them is to fight amongst each other. When you do that, you will see how things become much simpler. It is more of something that you tell them as your last wish. Tell them that fighting over finances isn't something you want them to do.

Important Milestones

You can speak about some significant milestones, telling your loved one where you wish to see them sometime down the road. You can tell them where you envision them, and you can also give them reasons for it. When you speak to your loved ones about where you see them, you can also tell them why you see potential in them and how they can grow to become great.

Last Rites

Speaking about last rites can be hard, especially when you are the one doing it yourself. So when talking to your loved ones, try to focus on speaking about how you'd want them to pay homage to you once you aren't there. How nice would it be to have things go your way? So you can speak to them about it and tell them why you think it is important.

Post Death Arrangements

Depending on what you want, you can speak to your loved ones about what kind of arrangement you want. Do you want a green burial, a traditional religious ceremony, a home funeral, or something else? Depending on your preferences, you can let your loved ones know about this so they can make arrangements accordingly. You can even have an alternate arrangement like serving your favorite food to those who come to mourn your loss. Doing these things really helps and can allow you to be at peace knowing that things will turn out the way you wanted.

Try to Get Peace

When you grow older, you must start focusing on mental peace. We often recommend that youngsters take care of their older parents or grandparents. However, it is equally important for every person getting older to take care of themselves physically and mentally. It is always best you calm your mind as much as possible. For that, there are many things you can do.

- **Religion**

You can get in touch with religious leaders who counsel you and make you understand things from another great perspective. Regardless of what religion you follow, when you focus on that, it can help you stay grounded and can help you see the good in things.

- **Support Groups**

There are many support groups that you can join. These can help you see through things properly. When others talk to you about their life experiences, it will help you make meaning of your life too. Speaking to those facing something similar can help you make more meaning of your own situation and help you understand love in the best way. People's lessons often make us learn things in a way we cannot recognize things ourselves.

- **Writing**

Many thoughts come to your head when you know you are nearing the end of your life. Sometimes, penning your thoughts down helps make you understand things more clearly. Sometimes, there are many things you don't want to talk about. When you pen those thoughts down, it allows you to understand them much better. Writing is a useful creative outlet that helps you to understand yourself well.

- **Spend Time with Your Loved Ones**

Surround yourself with as much love as you can. Spending time with those you love can be very soothing. It helps you understand things in a much better way. You get a lot of peace when you surround yourself with love and laughter. Do that as much as you can, and you will see how stress-free it makes you feel.

- **Do Not Depend On Others**

In order to have a peaceful life, one should not depend upon others. No matter how old or alone you get, you must find activities yourself so that you don't need to rely on others. People should never be the source of peace in anyone's life because, more or less, we all live by the choices we make. So, to avoid conflict with our loved ones, we should be well-equipped when it comes to loneliness and old age.

Medical Care

Thanks to modern medicine, several different ways can be used to help a person. Hence, it is important that you speak to your doctor about most things that you think matter. You can talk about all the options you see ahead of you and what kind of end-of-life support you want. Having agency and control over this is important, so you must make sure that you talk about it with the others first.

When nearing the end of life, you might need advanced medical care, especially if you are suffering from a chronic illness. You must let people around you know about medical care concerns. Many people wish to be in hospice instead of staying at the hospital. Some even have valid concerns about never being put on a ventilator, regardless of how worse their situations become. So if you have any reservations about medical care, make sure that you let others know about it. When you do that, you make sure you plan things according to your wants.

Do Things That Make a Difference

The cycle of life is as follows: we all are born, and then we live some years and leave for our final abode. But those who are gone aren't mostly always remembered. They live on in our memories for some time, and then we, too, tend to forget about them. So it is a great idea to do something that makes your legacy live on. When everything and everyone is easily elapsed, what can you do then?

- **Plant a Tree**

You can plant a tree in your name. When you do that, you are contributing to making the world a much better place; that is how your legacy can live on.

- **Contribute to a Good Cause**

You can even contribute to a positive cause. For example, if someone is building a shelter for animals, or an orphanage, you can contribute to that good cause. For as long as that cause lives, you will continue to live through that cause. When you do something like that, you positively contribute to the world, and then people remember you for your good deeds over time.

- **Find Your Way to Someone's Heart**

When you touch lives, you increase your chances of living in someone's heart even when you die. How do you do that? Maybe you could financially help someone who couldn't pay their medical bills? Maybe you could teach someone who was struggling with exams? Maybe you could be there for someone who was struggling in life. When you do these things, you allow yourselves to make your way to someone's heart. When you do so with genuine intent, they will remember you and will pray for you even when you aren't there.

So by bearing in mind all of these things, you can make the end of your life much easier. When you age, you get close to the end of your life. So when things are sorted out, you can be much more at peace knowing that things are going your way.

You can be at peace knowing you won't leave your loved ones to deal with your dealings. So it is always best that you plan way before time. Regardless of what stage of life you are at, start planning for the day that you won't be there. Remember that life is very uncertain. You don't have to be sick or very old to die. Life can take many turns when you least expect them, so you might as well be ready well before time.

Ongoing Scientific Research

There is a lot of ongoing research about aging, fighting off several health problems, and longevity. Scientists have been trying to find out how we can work on improving the quality of our lives while we age gracefully. There are so many diseases that still don't have a cure, like cancer. So many people die from cancer every year. With so much ongoing research about how we can fight off this disease, we still haven't been able to crack the code. Scientists worldwide are in a race to invent the miracle pill, but nothing has been able to help. So while we feel we are getting closer to humanity's dream of extreme life longevity, we don't really know the real situation or if we will ever get there.

The hunt for immorality got scientists to discover Costa Rica's blue zone. Several centenarians live in this zone, and male life expectancy is the highest here. The main reason is due to their healthy lifestyle. But scientists also believe that this is because of their DNA. The sections of DNA found at the end of chromosomes are longer than those of the average person. Scientists are trying to crack the code for the longevity of one's life but haven't been able to do so yet. While nothing is certain, and there is no proven method to increase your life span, a few tips can help increase your life expectancy.

Tips to Increase Life Expectancy

The average life expectancy in the world today is 73.4 years. You can work on your overall health with these general guidelines.

- **Focus on Nutrition**

Time and again, the importance of eating well has been focused upon in this book. The idea is to ensure that you have a balanced diet so your body gets food from all food groups. This allows you to remain healthy, which increases your chances of extending your life span. But this surely doesn't mean that you should overeat. Overeating can make you obese, which can cause a lot of issues for you. Your body must work harder to digest all that food, which can strip years of your life. So try to focus on eating in moderation. While it is alright to indulge once in a while, try always to eat healthy so that you can work on your body and your overall health.

- **Be Happy**

Being mentally healthy is extremely important. Being in a good place mentally allows you to live a great quality of life. For that, it is important that you are happy. So do things that make you happy. For example, if you like to spend time with your loved ones, do that. If you like being around nature, do that. Prioritize your happiness over all other things, and you will see how much it helps you just be yourself and focus on your life.

- **Quit Smoking**

Smoking is very bad for your lungs in the long run. You will be surprised to know how many years can be added to your life if you quit smoking. A research study shows that quitting smoking at the age of thirty could add around ten years to your life. Imagine how great that would be! So try to stop smoking at the earliest that you can. This can be hard because nicotine addiction is real. But if you try, you will surely be able to do it.

- **Quit Alcohol**

Alcohol is also known to have terrible effects on your body. So try to quit. Again, this can be very tough for people who are heavy drinkers. But you need to be one to decide what you want. You need to be one to decide how much your life matters to you.

So if you want to increase your life expectancy, try quitting alcohol. It will help you elongate your life span.

- **Get Enough Sleep**

There are several instances in this book where the importance of sleep has been stressed upon. In several instances, tips for better sleep have also been given. So try to get as much sleep as you can. This will surely help you improve the quality of your life. When you rest well, your body prepares itself to fight off diseases. This helps you increase your chances of living longer.

- **Shed Off Extra Weight**

Carrying extra weight is an added burden. Being overweight brings with it its own set of problems. You are more likely to suffer from diabetes and other health issues when overweight. So try to shed off those extra kilos to increase your chances of living longer. Focus on your nutrition and exercise regularly. This can help you get what you want, increasing your chances of living longer.

- **Get Spiritual**

Sometimes there are events in our life that bog us down. Certain things take a toll on our mental health as well. So dealing with that is something very important. For that, try focusing on being spiritual as much as possible. Connect with your inner self in any way that works for you. This can help you deal with your problems in a much better way. This surely doesn't mean that things won't bother you at all. But you will have a proven method to help you deal with those, eventually allowing you to increase your life span.

- **Forgive Others**

Very often, we hold grudges against people in our hearts. These are people who have wronged us. We find it very hard to forgive them because we can't just let go of how they hurt us at a certain point in life. When you let go of the grudges in your heart, you will see its proven health benefits. Extra stress is linked to heart disease, stroke, poor lung health, and blood pressure problems. So you must try to forgive others for working on your physical health, allowing you to improve the quality of your life.

- **Drive Safely**

Road accidents are one of the leading causes of early deaths worldwide. So whenever you are driving, try to be as cautious as possible. Not just that, but also try to have your safety gear on to ensure you don't get injured. Have your helmet on when you drive, and have the seatbelt on at all times. This will help you protect yourself in the case of an accident or an injury.

- **Don't Take Your Health Lightly**

If there are certain health problems you are facing, the last thing you should do is take that lightly. Instead, try to cater to all health issues as soon as possible. At any point in time in life, when you face health issues, try to deal with them well. See a doctor if you have to. Never ignore any sign that tells you something is wrong with your body. When you do that, the chances of the problem getting bigger are much higher, increasing your chances of more problems.

When you prioritize your health, you will see how much your life improves. This way, you will also be able to work on your health and increase your chances of living longer. While none of these tips are proven, they can all help you increase overall health benefits.

Way Forward

So now that you have ample knowledge about aging and all that comes with it, the idea is for you to understand that aging isn't a problem- it is a completely natural process. There is a specific life cycle that we all have to go through. We all have to grow old one day and realize that our bodies will change as we age. This means that we will see many changes in ourselves. Many a time, these changes will not be positive. We need to shape ourselves to understand how and why it is essential to deal with these changes.

Inculcating a more positive mindset is the most important thing. When you do that, you focus on the positive in life and take things lightly. Understand that your body will not function the same way for all times to come. Let nature run its course while you do your best to manage the process and age as gracefully as you can. Focus on what you can do- like eating well, exercising regularly, and engaging in healthy activities- then leave the rest up to fate. You will see how you make your life so much simpler when you do that.

The key here is to work on a more positive mindset, which eventually allows you to grow to become a better version of yourself.

Ways to Become a More Positive Person

Here are a few ways that you can train yourself to think positively. This will allow you to make the best use of this gift called life. Of course, how you look at your life depends entirely on your outlook. The way you think is what matters the most. So even if that doesn't come naturally to you, you can work on it and will surely see improvement with time.

- **Filtering**

Look at the negative aspects of a situation and try to filter them out first. When you make a conscious effort to filter that out, you will understand your life in a much better way. For example, if you had a bad day at work, try to let go of the negative feelings and focus on all the positive things that happened during the day. This shift in perspective and outlook will help you understand your life better, allowing you to live a much more fulfilled life.

- **Surround Yourself with Positive People**

The company you keep has a great effect on you and the way that you function. When you surround yourself with pessimistic people, you tend to take that approach to life, which is not suitable for you. So always try to have positive people around you. When you do that, you will see how the positivity spreads, allowing you to become a happier and healthier version of yourself. Negative people can be toxic and only focus on the bad in life. When you surround yourself with such people, you tend to adopt the same approach, which is not the right thing to do. Life is very short, so surround yourself with inspiring people who help you see the good in situations, even when things are not working out your way.

- **Open Yourself Up to Humor**

Being jovial is always a good idea. It helps you take things lightly and allows you to see the positive in different situations. So always keep yourself open to humor. When you do that, you can greatly lower your stress levels and anxiety. It allows you to keep yourself happy.

- **Practice Gratitude**

This book talks about the importance of practicing gratitude in several places. First, practicing gratitude allows you to see the good in things. It allows you to be grateful for whatever you have been given. Keeping a gratitude journal can help too. Set aside time to look at all you have been blessed with each day. This will help you have a much more positive outlook on life, allowing you to become a much better version of yourself.

- **Stop Comparing**

More often than not, we compare our lives to those around us. This has especially become more prevalent in the era of social media, where we tend to be extremely focused on what others are doing. This is detrimental to your mental health and only makes you focus on what others have and don't. So always focus on what you have, and never compare your life to someone else's. We each live unique lives and have our own things to look forward to. Unfavorable comparisons with other people only make us feel worse about ourselves. So that is something we need to avoid under all circumstances.

- **Be Kind**

Be nice to others around you. When you are nice to other people, it makes you feel much better on the inside. It gives you a positive outlook and allows you to see the good in things. Knowing that you made someone feel good only makes you feel better. So try to always focus on that. Maybe you could bake a cake for a loved one on their birthday or buy something for someone who can't afford it. When you put a smile on someone else's face, you understand the true meaning of happiness.

- **Celebrate the Little Things**

Every little thing that happens and makes you happy calls for a celebration. Never wait for the big moments to celebrate. When you celebrate the littlest of things, it will allow you to see the good in life. It will enable you to understand that there is no better way to live than to be happy with minor accomplishments. This is your life, and only you can make it better. So to have a more positive outlook on life, be focused on the good.

- **Practice Mindfulness**

Practicing mindfulness every day allows you to unwind and relax, even when things aren't working out your way. So try to set some time aside every day to practice mindfulness. This will only make you feel much better and help you change your outlook. Stress reduction is one of the major aspects of thinking positively. So when you do that, you will see how much better your life automatically becomes.

- **Follow a Healthy Lifestyle**

This book is all about having a healthy lifestyle. It has many different things that it focuses on, like nutrition, exercise, and stress reduction. So try to focus on having a healthy lifestyle by doing all that is needed to help you get one. When you are healthy within, it also shows up on the outside, allowing you to live a fulfilled life.

When you consciously follow all of these tips, you will see how much better your life becomes. A positive outlook on life allows you to see the good in things. It allows you to age gracefully. We all have to age, so we'd much rather do it with a smile rather than lament the times that have already passed.

Morgan Harper Nichols says, "One day, you will look back and see that all along you were blooming." I love this quote because it focuses on your mindset. Only when you focus on having a positive mindset will you see the good in things. You will only see how you were blooming when you focus on all you have achieved. Wisdom comes with age too. With numerous years of experience, you become much wiser.

If you have people living with you wanting to benefit from your wisdom, then there is nothing better than passing it all on. Remember, age with a smile and gratitude in your heart, and you will see life as nothing short of a gift from God. Happiness lies within; it is only we who have to unmask it.

Bibliography

PRB, 2022. *Countries With the Oldest Populations in the World.* [Online]

Available at: https://www.prb.org/resources/countries-with-the-oldest-populations-in-the world/#:~:text=Asia%20and%20Europe%20are%20home,at%20 just%20under%2022%20percent.

Berger, S., 2021. *10 Pieces Of Expert Nutrition Advice For 2022.* [Online]

Available at: https://www.forbes.com/health/body/expert-nutrition-advice/

Fegerberg, P., 2021. Fast Eating Is Associated with Increased BMI among High-School Students. *Nutrients.*

News, 2016. *10 COMMON ELDERLY HEALTH ISSUES.* [Online]
Available at: https://vitalrecord.tamhsc.edu/10-common-elderly-health-issues/

Wong, C. W., 2015. Vitamin B12 deficiency in the elderly: is it worth screening? *Hong Kong Med J.*